# Antibiotic Resistance:

# An Emerging Pandemic

# Antibiotic Resistance:
# An Emerging Pandemic

Written & Edited by:

Dr. Austin Mardon, Hafsa Alamagan, Christina MacDonald, Julia Cara, Jasrita Singh, Maryam Oloriegbe, Gurman Barara, Tolu Atama, Amy Li, Sriraam Sivachandran, Margaret Wa Yan Choi & Suad Alad

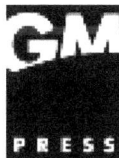

**GM**
PRESS

Cover and typeset by A. Boyd

Paperback ISBN 978-1-77369-241-8

Ebook ISBN 978-1-77369-238-8

Golden Meteorite Press
103 11919 82 St NW
Edmonton, AB T5B 2W3
www.goldenmeteoritepress.com

# Chapter 1: History of Antibiotics

By: Dr. Austin Mardon & Christina MacDonald

## Introduction

Widely considered one of the most notable discoveries of the 20th century, antibiotics changed the medical world by providing new ways to combat infections. Unfortunately, with the increased discovery and use of antibiotics came a new issue: antibiotic resistance. Before delving into antibiotic resistance and its implications, one must better understand the history of antibiotic discovery.

## Definitions and some key terminology

## What are antibiotics?

To begin to understand the realm of antibiotics, one must be familiar with the term microorganism. Breaking down the term, a microorganism can be understood as a very small (micro), living entity (organism) that is only visible under a microscope.

This includes bacteria, fungi, and viruses. It is important to note that while viruses are not technically alive, they can be considered microorganisms due to their ability to infect host cells and replicate (National Cancer Institute, n.d.). Understanding this in terms of antibiotics is important because antibiotics are defined as substances or drugs that combat bacterial infections (Nicolaou & Rigol, 2017). In other words, antibiotics attack microorganisms. Another term, often used interchangeably with antibiotics is 'antimicrobial' or 'antimicrobial agents'. These are umbrella terms that include antibiotics as they work against (anti) other microbes (microorganisms), in this case, bacteria.

According to the Oxford English Dictionary, an antibiotic is "injurious to or destructive of living matter, [especially] microorganisms" (OED Online, 2021). This definition is rooted in the term 'antibiose' or 'antibiosis', credited to microbiologist Jean Paul Vuillemin in 1890. He defined antibiose as the opposite of symbiosis or, in other words, when a living organism kills a different living organism for survival purposes (Durand et al., 2019).

Moreover, the Oxford English Dictionary defines an antibiotic substance as "one of a class of substances produced by living organisms and capable of destroying or inhibiting the growth of microorganisms; [specifically] any of these substances for therapeutic purposes" (OED Online, 2021). Microorganisms naturally produce substances to fight off other microorganisms, making it likely that, as Vuillemin alluded to, the natural production of antibiotics serves as a survival mechanism enabling microorganisms to protect themselves and to prey upon their natural competition (Durand et al., 2019; Hutchings et al., 2019).

## Gram-positive and gram-negative bacteria

Although antibiotics have similar overall purposes, they do not all target the same bacteria. In literature, there is often reference to gram-positive and gram-negative bacteria. What is important to understand is that the cell envelope composition of various bacteria differs, so depending on the antibiotic, it may or may not be able to penetrate the bacteria's specific structure (Silhavy et al., 2010). Gram-positive bacteria have no outer membrane, but are instead surrounded by many thick layers of sugars and amino acids (the smallest unit of proteins) that form what is called peptidoglycan layers. With gram-negative bacteria, this wall of peptidoglycan is thin, but it is surrounded by an outer membrane of large molecules of lipids and complex sugars (referred to as polysaccharides) (Silhavy et al., 2010). The differences in cell composition require different antibiotics to break them down.

## Natural, semi-synthetic and fully synthetic antibiotics

It should also be noted that antibiotics can be natural or synthetic. Natural antibiotics are produced from microorganisms, for example, mold and organisms in soil. Synthetic antibiotics are either semi-synthetic or fully chemically synthetic, meaning they are partially or fully chemically engineered in a lab (Demain, 2009).

Natural products do not need human involvement to exist. Semisynthesis occurs when pre-existing structures are modified after fermentation has occurred—fermentation being a chemical breakdown process (Ribeiro da Cunha et al., 2019). Fully synthetic antibiotics are chemically related to natural antibiotics, but can be made efficiently for clinical use (Ribeiro da Cunha et al., 2019).

With a clearer understanding of some important terms, the following sections will explore the timeline of some significant antibiotic discoveries that have led to current drugs and concerns with antibiotic resistance.

## Where it all started: The first known uses and discoveries of antibiotics

Antibiotic use can be traced back thousands of years to countries such as Egypt, China, and Greece—notably, to remedies using bread mold and soil with medicinal (antibiotic) properties (Hutchings et al., 2019). Notably, the year 1640 marked one of the first times bread mold was recorded as an agent to fight against infections (Gould, 2016).

There was much speculation about the transmission of infection and some evidence indicating bacteria could cause infection. In the early 1800s, Jakob Henle hypothesized that infection could be transferred from the sick to the healthy. The first person to successfully be able to prove that a specific agent (bacteria) was correlated to a disease was Robert Koch, a German physician (Mohr, 2016). He was able to identify specific agents of disease for infections such as cholera and tuberculosis. He also was the inventor of a staining dye that led to the dyes used in laboratories today (Mohr, 2016). His hypotheses and discoveries involving bacteria as a causal agent for disease serve as a pivotal point in the history of antibiotic discovery.

Fast-forward to the end of the 19th century, Jean Paul Vuillemin is associated with the initial use of the term 'antibiose' in the late 1800s. Only a few years later, in 1893, the first nature-derived antibiotic, called mycophenolic acid, was discovered by Italian physician Bartolomeo Gosio. However, some sources may not report this as the first natural antibiotic discovery as mycophenolic acid was not widely known until it was rediscovered in 1913 in the United States (Nicolaou & Rigol, 2017). Furthermore, its structure was not fully discovered until the early 1950s and it was only able to be fully synthesized by the end of the 1960s (Nicolaou & Rigol, 2017).

## The first modern antibiotic: Salvarsan

Salvarsan, also known as arsphenamine or compound 606, is a discovery accredited to German physician Paul Ehrlich and was approved for use in 1910. It is considered to be the first synthetic (human-made) antimicrobial agent used clinically (Nicolaou & Rigol, 2017; Hutchings et al, 2019). Deriving the drug from arsenic, Ehrlich paved the road to modern chemotherapy using dye experimentation to show the impacts the drug had on specifically stained cells (Mohr, 2016).

Salvarsan was used to treat syphilis, a sexually transmitted bacterial infection that presents itself as sores during the early stages but can become increasingly severe to the point that it results in organ damage and death (CDC, 2017).

## Prontosil: a synthetic sulfa drug

Sulfa drugs, or sulfonamides are the first class of antibiotics to be discovered. The discovery is accredited to Gerhard Domagk, a German physician who, following the lead of Paul Ehrlich, used dyes to stain target bacteria (Hutchings et al., 2019). These drugs bind to sites on bacteria that are critical for the formation of important nutrients, inhibiting proper function (National Institutes of Health, 2012). They present bacteriostatic effects on various gram-positive bacteria, and a few types of gram-negative bacteria (Mohr, 2016).

A notable drug in this category, Prontosil, marked another great triumph in the history of antibiotics. Prontosil entered the market in 1935 and had extremely positive impacts on fatalities due to pneumonia and meningitis—a lung infection and inflammation that causes swelling in the membranes around the brain and spinal cord, respectively (Mohr, 2016).

## The accidental discovery of penicillin revolutionized antibiotic discovery

One of the most popular antibiotic discoveries is that of penicillin. Alexander Fleming, a Scottish scientist, happened upon his discovery of penicillin accidentally after returning from a vacation in September of 1928. In his writings, Fleming (1929) recounts that, upon his return, he found one of the bacteria he was studying was contaminated with mold. He observed that the mold seemed to cause the disintegration of the bacterial cells it was closest to; the bacterial colonies were less affected the farther they were from the mold. This led him to conclude that something in the mold killed the bacteria (Nicolaou & Rigol, 2017).

Despite being an accident, the discovery of penicillin became very important, especially during World War II where it was used to aid in the treatment of wounded soldiers (Nicolaou & Rigol, 2017). Mass production followed this success, leading to penicillin being nicknamed 'the wonder drug' (Microbiology Society, 2015).

Penicillin, a gram-positive bacteria attacker, is still widely used today. However, rather than being popular amongst soldiers in battle, it is associated with the treatment of various bacterial infections including respiratory tract infections as well as mouth, throat, and ear infections (U.S. National Library of Medicine, 2021).

There have been many subsequent discoveries of antibiotics in the family of penicillin. According to the CDC (2014), one of the most commonly prescribed antibiotics is amoxicillin, which belongs to the penicillin family.

Although there have been a multitude of advancements in the study of antibiotics, Fleming's discovery of penicillin remains one of the most prominent and revolutionary discoveries in the history of antibiotic development.

## Actinomycetes: An important discovery for the

## world of antibiotics

Selman Waksman provided a well-cited definition of the word antibiotic, stating that it "is a chemical substance, produced by microorganisms, which has the capacity to inhibit the growth of and even to destroy bacteria and other microorganisms" (Waksman, 1947).

In addition to this popular definition, Waksman significantly contributed to furthering antibiotic history. He identified actinomycetes, essential microorganisms that exist in the soil that are crucial for natural well-being and have been prime contributors to the discovery of novel antibiotics (Hutchings et al., 2019; Genilloud, 2010). Actinomycetes can be linked to over 10,000 bacterial compounds and antibiotics such as streptomycin, tetracycline, erythromycin, and vancomycin because they all come from chemical reactions of actinomycetes —specifically from actinomycetes' secondary metabolism (Weber et al., 2015).

## The discovery of streptomycin marks another milestone in antibiotic discovery

Just as there are many different microorganisms with various structures, various antibiotics have different microorganisms they target. Penicillin resistant bacteria was discovered in 1940, so the discovery of streptomycin in 1943 by Albert Schatz and Selman Waksman was an important advancement in the realm of antibiotics as it was able to target types of microorganisms that penicillin could not; namely, gram-negative bacteria (Hutchings et al., 2019; Nicolaou & Rigol, 2017). In addition, streptomycin is able to inhibit bacterial growth, essentially leading to bacterial cell death (Nicolaou & Rigol, 2017). Notably, streptomycin served to treat tuberculosis, an infectious bacterial disease affecting the lungs and potentially other body organs (CDC, 2016).

Streptomycin was the first discovered antibiotic in the aminoglycoside class. This class of antibiotics is considered a broad-spectrum group of antibiotics as they can target a wide range of infections but are predominantly used against gram-negative bacteria (Mohr, 2016; Germovesek et al., 2017).

# The 'golden age' of antibiotics

The 'Golden Age' of antibiotics occurred in the 20th century, around the 1940s or 1950s, and came to an end in the 1960s (Nicolaou & Rigol, 2017; Davies, 2006). Following the discovery of penicillin, there was a rush to identify new natural sources that could serve as antibiotics. With a seemingly newfound fervour for antibiotic discovery, half of the antibiotic drugs we know today were discovered within a 20 year period (Davies, 2006).

A few important discoveries will be explored in further detail: chloramphenicol, tetracyclines, erythromycins and vancomycin.

## Chloramphenicol

Chloramphenicol is the first natural antibiotic that could be chemically synthesized rather than undergo the natural fermentation process (Nicolaou & Rigol, 2017).

Chloramphenicol was discovered by both John Ehrlich in 1947 and soon after by David Gottlieb; these discoveries were independent. Chloramphenicol works to inhibit protein formation in bacterial cells (Mohr, 2016). This antibiotic gained great recognition when it was used against epidemic typhus, a bacterial infection spread by infected lice (CDC, 2020). Once the drug was fully synthesized, it became the best-selling drug for a period of time (Nicolaou & Rigol, 2017).

In today's society, chloramphenicol can be prescribed as drops to treat various infections of the eye, for example conjunctivitis (also known as pink eye); it can also be used to treat ear infections (NHS, 2018b).

## Tetracyclines

Considered to be one of the most important classes of antibiotics, tetracyclines are able to attack both gram-positive and gram-negative bacteria, disabling the bacterial cells from being able to function properly, grow, or replicate (Nicolaou & Rigol, 2017; Chopra & Roberts, 2001). For this reason, tetracyclines are considered to have bacteriostatic effects.

The first tetracycline, known as chlortetracycline was discovered by Benjamin M. Duggar, an American plant physiologist, in 1948 (Nicolaou & Rigol, 2017). Since then, there have been many different natural, semi-synthetic, and chemically synthesized tetracyclines discovered.

One antibiotic in the tetracycline class that is in current use is doxycycline. It is used to treat various chest, skin, and sexually transmitted infections (NHS, 2018c).

## Erythromycins

Members of this group of antibiotics (erythromycin A and B) were isolated from a soil sample— brought from the Philippines to the United States—by a group of scientists led by James M. McGuire in 1952. Depending on the strain of erythromycin, it can inhibit the growth and reproduction of bacteria, or it can kill the bacteria—in other words, they can have bacteriostatic or bactericidal effects (Nicolaou & Rigol, 2017). Being able to fight against both gram-negative and gram-positive bacteria, erythromycin was traditionally used to treat numerous types of infections, including respiratory infections as well as prevent newborns from getting conjunctivitis (pink eye) (Farzam et al., 2020).

Within the erythromycin group falls azithromycin, one of the most commonly prescribed antibiotics in the United States in 2014 (CDC, 2014). This antibiotic is prescribed to treat infections of the chest, nose and throat such as pneumonia and sinus infections. It can also treat skin infections, Lyme disease and some sexually transmitted infections (NHS, 2018a).

## Vancomycin

Vancomycin was appropriately named for its capacity to 'vanish' bacteria. This antibiotic falls within a larger family of antibiotics called glycopeptides and was found in 1953 in soil from the Southeast Asian island of Borneo. It acts against gram-positive bacteria as well as penicillin-resistant bacteria (Nicolaou & Rigol, 2017). In the years following its discovery, vancomycin was approved and used to treat bacterial infections, but due to high levels of toxicity, it's popularity decreased.

Even though it was originally discovered in the early 1950s, full synthesis was only accomplished in 1999 (Nicolaou & Rigol, 2017). In current times, vancomycin is used to treat colitis—intestinal inflammation due to bacteria (U.S. National Library of Medicine, 2016).

## A review of some notable discoveries: Nobel Prize winners

The following list highlights Nobel Prizes awarded for some of the great milestones in the history of antibiotic discoveries:

Robert Koch won the Nobel Prize in Physiology or Medicine in 1905 for his contribution to the understanding of tuberculosis.

Paul Ehrlich and Ilya Ilyich Mechnikov were awarded the Nobel Prize in Physiology or Medicine in 1908 for their work in immunity (Salvarsan).

Gerhard Domagk was awarded the Nobel Prize in Physiology or Medicine in 1939 for his discovery of Prontosil.

Sir Alexander Fleming along with Ernst Boris Chain and Sir Howard Walter Florey won the Nobel Prize in Physiology or Medicine in 1945 for their discovery of penicillin.

Selman Abraham Waksman won the Nobel Prize for Physiology or Medicine in 1952 for the discovery of streptomycin (The Nobel Prize, 2021).

## The 'golden age' of antibiotics is long over

During the 'Golden Age' of antibiotic discovery, there was a rapid increase in knowledge of different antibiotic-producing organisms, but now there are less rapid advances as many soils have been tested. With a low yield of novel antibiotics from natural products, discoveries of new classes of antibiotics are scarce. However, there is still some potential for progress as new environments, such as marine environments, become accessible through novel technologies. Moreover, scientists can now look at how different bacteria are co-evolving as well as at new technologies that allow for a more in-depth understanding of the human microbiome to further their studies (Hutchings et al., 2019).

The use of antibiotics is still quite high as data from the Government of Canada (2019) reported over 24 million prescriptions filled for antibiotics in 2017 alone . The large issue that then arises is that in the decades following the 'Golden Age', there has been a lull in the development of novel antibiotics simultaneous with a significant increase in antibiotic resistance (Gould, 2016).

The following chapters will further explore the concept of antibiotics, examining the current implications of this era of antibiotic resistance.

# Chapter 2: Origins and Evolution of Antibiotic Resistance

By: Dr. Austin Mardon & Julia Cara

## What is Antibiotic Resistance?

Antibacterial resistance is an evolutionary survival response to the use of antibiotics and occurs when bacteria evolve in such a way that they no longer respond to medication (WHO, 2020). Just like other organisms, bacteria evolve over time. In addition, environmental factors like resource availability determine the survival of bacterial populations, and so bacteria are also subjected to the whims of Darwin's natural selection. Thus, the success of existing and future antibiotics depends on the target bacteria's capacity to adapt and develop tolerance to the therapy at hand.

Antibiotic resistance was first described in the late 1930s, shortly after sulfonamides – one of the first effective antimicrobials – was synthesized in 1931. The first clinical use of sulfonamides to treat streptococcal infections was reported in 1933 when the drug was administered to a boy dying of staphylococcal septicemia and he miraculously recovered (Shambaugh, 1966). However, sulfonamide resistance was described shortly thereafter. Similarly, mutant strains of Mycobacterium tuberculosis were reported shortly after streptomycin was introduced to treat tuberculosis in 1944 (Davies & Davies, 2010).

Penicillin, discovered by Alexander Fleming in 1928, did not become widely used as an antibiotic until the mid to late 1940s. However, bacteria had already begun building a tolerance towards the life-saving medicine as early as 1940 when Abraham and Chain reported finding a bacterial enzyme capable of destroying penicillin (Abraham & Chain, 1940). This enzyme was called bacterial penicillinase (Davies & Davies, 2010). As penicillin rose to prominence in medicine it was hailed as a miracle drug and used to treat infections like meningitis and pneumonia. However, with increased use more and more resistant strains arose. In 1945, shortly after winning a Nobel Prize for his discovery, Alexander Fleming himself warned that the "public will demand [the drug and] … then will begin an era … of abuses" (Ventola, 2015).

The first penicillin-resistant bacterial strain was Staphylococcus aureus, which can cause skin, bone, and heart valve infections, as well as pneumonia. It was discovered in 1942, only a year after penicillin was formally approved for use (CDC, 2020). Then, penicillin-resistant strains of Streptococcus pneumoniae and Neisseria gonorrhoeae (which cause pneumonia and gonorrhea, respectively) were discovered in 1967 and 1976.

In fact, the discovery of resistant strains of bacteria has become a recurring pattern in antibiotic discovery. Bacteria are highly resilient and capable of adaptation. Ever since the discovery of penicillin and the subsequent discovery of penicillin-resistant germs, scientists have been playing a game of cat and mouse as they try to outsmart the ever-evolving bacteria. With each new antibiotic discovery comes a newly identified resistant germ. Sometimes the strains take decades to develop resistance. Such is the case with amphotericin B, which was first released in 1959 (CDC, 2020). The amphotericin B-resistant Candida auris germ strain (which can cause blood and ear infections in hospitalized patients) was not identified until 2016. Other strains are identified almost immediately. For example, methicillin-resistant Staphylococcus aureus was reported in 1960, the same year the Methicillin drug was released. Though these drugs are still used today and are effective against many bacteria, the emergence of resistant bacterial strains is of great concern.

## How Resistance Emerges

Resistance emerges by mutation and natural selection. Like all other organisms, bacterial reproduction can result in genetic mutations, some of which are negligent while others improve the bacteria's ability to survive.

Consider a population of bacteria which is genetically diverse. The introduction of antibiotics to this population might kill off most of these bacteria – namely those that are most susceptible to the antibiotic's mechanisms of action. However, some bacteria will survive due to variations in their genetics. That resistant bacterial population now has access to more of the resources it needs to survive and reproduce (nutrients and environment), has fewer competitors, and is, therefore, in a position to thrive.

When these resistant bacteria repopulate the area, the next round of antibiotics will become less effective. The antibiotics might still kill some of the bacteria – those that are weaker, or perhaps have developed a mutation that negatively affects their chance for survival – but those that remain after the second round of antibiotics will be even more resistant.

Antibacterial resistance can also be achieved by transferring genetic material between organisms, a process termed 'horizontal gene transfer'. In its essence, horizontal gene transfer allows resistant bacteria to share their 'knowledge' with other bacteria. Genes which carry information about resistance (instructions about how to destroy or avoid antibiotics) are often found within plasmids – small fragments of DNA which can be absorbed or 'taken up' by bacteria. Once absorbed, the bacteria can use this genetic information to make antibiotic-resistant modifications to their own cells (Wright, 2012).

Combining the ideas of mutation and horizontal gene transfer, one can see how the challenge of antibiotic resistance grows. Though most horizontally acquired genes cause deleterious (negative) or neutral effects to the recipient's chromosomal DNA, the spread of even just one or two advantageous mutations via horizontal gene transfer can render an entire population of bacteria resistant to a certain drug (Thomas, 2005).

A helpful analogy is to compare bacteria to human immune cells. When a pathogen enters the body, the immune system launches a coordinated response. After immune cells encounter and successfully destroy a pathogen, surviving immune cells form memory B cells which store information about the pathogen and defense strategy. This information can be 'remembered' and used to inform future immune responses should that same pathogen be encountered again. Similarly, bacteria which survive an antibiotic 'attack', or which undergo an advantageous mutation gain immunity and share this information with other bacteria to increase their chances of survival should they encounter more antibiotics. As this cycle continues, the bacteria's resistance to antibiotics will strengthen.

As Harvard Medical School Professor Christopher T. Walsh states in his textbook Antibiotics: Challenges, Mechanisms, Opportunities, "Resistance is not a matter of if but only of when". He warns of two consequences of antibiotic use: firstly, that the lifetime of any widely used antibiotic is finite, and secondly, that there will always be a need for new antibiotics to treat the resistant bacterial populations that form after initial antibiotic treatment (Walsh, 2016).

## Contributing Factors

A driving factor in the emergence of antibiotic resistance is the overuse of broad-spectrum antibiotics. For many years, general antibiotics were prescribed for bacterial infections ranging from a small cut on the hand to severe sepsis or tuberculosis. The overuse of antibiotics for lesser-severity, easily resolvable wounds lead to multi-drug resistant bacterial pathogens such as Staphylococcus aureus. Antibiotics also kill beneficial bacteria which protect the body from infection, therefore antibiotics are both a cure and a cause of infection, depending on how they are used.

Surprisingly, incorrect prescriptions are as much to blame as overuse. Many of these erroneous prescriptions are ordered and used in hospital intensive care units (ICU). Surveillance data indicates that "30% to 60% of antibiotics prescribed in ICUs are unnecessary, inappropriate, or suboptimal" (Luyt, 2014). Unfortunately, barriers exist to lowering this number including the limited time and expertise of intensive care physicians, the severity of infections and the fragility of patients.

A third driving factor is the widespread use of antibiotics, not only geographically but functionally. Though traditionally considered a human medicine, antibiotics are used in agriculture. In 2016 approximately 70% of all medically important antibiotics in the United States were sold for intended use on animals (Dall, 2016). Antibiotics are used on animals to control disease, but also to improve the animals' metabolism and reduce the amount of food that is necessary to provide – all by promoting the growth of specific microbes that produce vitamins, amino acids, and other nutrients.

Unfortunately, using antibiotics for non-therapeutic uses has been proven to increase antibiotic resistance in pathogenic bacteria in the animals, animal-based food products, and the environment – air, soil and water – surrounding farms and animal factories (Dall, 2016).

## Antibiotic Cycling and Antibiotic Mixing

Hospitals are a key breeding ground for antibiotic resistance. Antibiotics are prescribed every day – necessary for infection control in post-op surgeries, cancer patients with chemotherapy-weakened immune systems, and for a variety of other reasons. Many approaches have been invented to tackle this issue in hospital settings, including antibiotic cycling and antibiotic mixing – both of which aim to "reduce the selective pressure for resistance" and protect the effectiveness of drugs (Dall, 2018).

First introduced in the 1980s, antibiotic cycling involves administering two or more antibiotic drugs (of different classes but similar strength) consecutively and in a cyclic pattern (Dall, 2018). Each antibiotic must be used for the same set period of time and is administered to every patient in need of antibiotics in a certain hospital ward. The hypothesis is that prescribing the same medicine to every patient and switching between types of antibiotics will prevent the often-rapid spread of multi-drug resistant bacteria between patients in hospital wards (Dall, 2018). This approach is often compared to the crop-rotation practice in farming which is meant to improve the health of soil by planting different crops every year; a practice which preserves rich nutrients and prevents weeds and pests. Similarly, it was hoped that if a population of bacteria didn't encounter a certain antibiotic during the time that that antibiotic was in the "off" stage of the cycle, then perhaps it would prevent resistant genes from being passed down during replication (bacterial reproduction) because the fitness costs of being drug-resistant would be too high (Beardmore, 2017).

Antibiotic mixing, despite its misleading name, does not refer to giving a mixture of several different antibiotics to a single patient – that is a separate practice called combination therapy. Instead, antibiotic mixing involves treating every patient on a hospital ward with a different antibiotic, effectively randomizing which medicine is given (Beardmore, 2017). Despite the data from clinical trials nearing 4 million patient-days of treatment (patient-days or person-days being a measurement of time used in clinical studies), there is still no conclusive evidence to deem either approach as particularly 'successful', much less point to a stronger option between them (Beardmore, 2017).

## Response to Antibiotic Resistance

The period of time between the early 1960s and late 1990s, colloquially referred to as the 'lean years' in antibiotic discovery due to a dramatic reduction in new antibiotic development, antibiotic resistance increased exponentially (Davies & Davies, 2010). During this time scientists worked to improve their understanding of antibiotic resistance through both pharmacological and biochemical means.

The knowledge gleaned from these studies informed attempts to negate the neutralizing abilities of resistant bacterial strains via chemical modification of existing drugs. Originally, antibiotics were natural products synthesized by microorganisms that had an effect on other microorganisms (Foster, 2017). Today, the broader classification of antibiotics includes both naturally occurring organic products, entirely synthetic molecules, and chemically modified antibiotics.

Chemical modifications made to naturally occurring antibiotic molecules include those meant to "increase potency, improve solubility and pharmacokinetics, and evade resistance mechanisms" (Foster, 2017). One such experiment was to chemically modify penicillin to prevent cleavage by penicillinases, which are bacterial enzymes capable of inactivating penicillin (Davies & Davies, 2010). Another experiment modified the nitrogen group in sulphanilamide to produce more effective chemical variants, of which sulfamethoxazole and sulfadiazine are still used clinically (Foster, 2017). In fact, both sulfamethoxazole and sulfadiazine are on the World Health Organization's Model List of Essential Medicines (WHO, 2019).

More recently, chemical modifications to existing antibiotics are being tailored to target specific bacteria based on the active site that the drug binds to (Foster, 2017). This targeted approach is part of a greater push to slow the evolution of new resistant strains by narrowing the spectrum of use of specific antibodies and targeting known pathogens instead of all bacteria (Wencewicz, 2018).

These modifications were meant to combat antibiotic resistance and supplement the dwindling pipeline of new medications at the time. Though many worked as intended, nature ultimately prevails, and bacteria has continued to find new ways to evade medical treatment.

## Superbugs and Staphylococcus aureus

Even more concerning is the fact that certain strains of bacteria have developed resistance to multiple antibacterial drugs over time. Take Staphylococcus aureus for example, which has proven itself highly capable of resisting antibiotics. Over the past 80 years it has developed antibiotic resistance to four different drugs: Penicillin in 1942, Methicillin in 1960, Vancomycin in 2002, and Daptomycin in 2004 (CDC, 2020).

Multi-drug resistant bacterial strains have, in recent years, become colloquially referred to as 'superbugs'. With multiple advantageous mutations, superbugs have increased morbidity, virulence, and mortality rates than other bacteria and present an urgent and deadly health crisis (Davies & Davies, 2010). Treating multi-drug resistant infections is becoming extraordinarily difficult. M. tuberculosis, described by Davies & Davies as "the archetypical human pathogen" for its continued evolution alongside medical advances, is another example of an extremely antibiotic-resistant disease. Infecting a third of the human population, there exists strains of M. tuberculosis that are entirely drug-resistant (Davies & Davies, 2010).

Superbugs represent the pinnacle of antibiotic resistance and the onset of the eventuality that scientists have been trying to put off for decades – the time when antibiotics will no longer work to fight off disease.

## Why is Antibiotic Resistance an Urgent Public Health Threat?

Antibiotic resistance does not only directly affect human health by hindering treatment of fatal diseases, but it also affects the veterinary and agriculture industries (CDC, 2020). Antibiotic use in agriculture and animal farming has resulted in antibiotic resistance in animals in the same fashion as we saw in humans. The antibiotic-resistant bacteria is highly transmissible, both to humans through dietary uptake and to the environment through animal waste products, and may be pathogenic to humans (Manyi-Loh, 2018). In the US alone, 2.8 million people become infected with antibiotic-resistant bacteria or fungi every year, with more than 35,000 related deaths (CDC, 2020).

The loss of effective antibiotics would be catastrophic to our society. Not only would we lose the ability to treat infections that arise from surgeries like joint replacements and organ transplants, but would lose the ability to treat common infections like strep throat and some sexually transmitted infections. We would also become vulnerable in fights against water and animal-borne diseases such as Lyme disease, Salmonella, tetanus, and gangrene.

Antibiotics are essential to medicine. They've been used since ancient times, with one of the first recorded usages of mold to treat infections dating back to 1640 (Gould, 2016). When penicillin was discovered it was heralded as a "miracle medicine". In fact, the discovery of antibiotics is arguably the most significant development in the history of medicine. The loss of this invention to antibiotic resistance and the emergence of "superbugs" threatens modern medicine and everyone on the planet.

# Chapter 3: Nearing the Return to a Pre-Antibiotic Era? Growing Threat of Antibiotic Resistance

By: Dr. Austin Mardon & Jasrita Singh

Antibacterial resistance is a silent, slowly growing tsunami that has the potential of sweeping away the foundation of modern medicine. The expansion of the resistome is imperiling the efficacy of antibiotics against infectious diseases, which threatens a potential return to the challenges of the pre-antibiotic era. This ever-growing problem is rooted in the rapid division of bacteria that survive post-antibiotic treatment, resulting in the subsequent transfer of resistance genes to their progeny. The serendipitous discovery of the first antibiotic by Alexander Fleming in 1928 set the paradigm for antibiotic discovery in the twentieth century. Owing to the armamentarium of antibiotics being developed during that time, many infectious disease specialists and medical doctors believed that bacterial infections could have been conquered. Three decades later, this optimism has fizzled out, our weapons are depleting and bacterial defences are becoming exponentially stronger. The last novel antibiotic class developed and approved for clinical use by the Food and

Drug Administration (FDA) was nearly three decades ago - in the 1980s. This lack of success in antibiotic discovery, coupled with the relentless rise in bacterial resistance, has led to the World Health Organization (WHO) declaring Antimicrobial Resistance (AMR) as one of the top ten global public health threats facing humanity.

Currently, AMR claims over 750,000 lives each year, with statistical models strongly suggesting over 10 million deaths annually by 2050. As a reference, this is 2 million more deaths than those estimated to occur from cancer each year. Currently, according to the WHO, tuberculosis is one of the top 10 causes of death globally. In 2019, an estimated 10 million people contracted TB and a total of 1.4 million people died from it. Multidrug-resistant tuberculosis and extensively drug-resistant tuberculosis are tuberculosis pathogenic strains that are resistant to anti-tuberculosis drugs. Infections from the two strains were responsible for approximately 214,000 deaths in 2018 and with growing resistance and the current level of effort, this number is expected to exponentially increase. In less than a decade, by 2030, up to 24 million people globally could be forced into extreme poverty as a result of antimicrobial resistance. This devastation may be averted with the discovery of novel drugs, however with the financially and temporally extensive decade-long discovery process, time is running out. We are standing on the precipice of a post-antibiotic era and if these predictions become a reality, not only will modern medicine will be gravely impacted, but it will pose one of the greatest public health challenges of the century and will be accompanied by major economic costs.

## Threat to Modern Medicine

The advent of antibiotics revolutionized medicine and clinical practices, and have served as "wonder drugs" in saving lives. Prior to the beginning of the 20th century, communicable infectious diseases were the leading cause of morbidity and mortality globally. Today, antibiotics have enabled the transition of the leading cause of death in the developed world from communicable infectious diseases to non-communicable diseases. The average life expectancy has dramatically increased from about mid 30s in the 1800s to mid 70s in 2019. Back then, the death of infants and children under 5 were widespread and today, most deaths occur amongst the elderly. This major stride is largely attributed to the discovery of drugs, like antibiotics, for battling infectious diseases. The 19th century was characterized by the persistent and rampant spread of lethal infectious diseases including smallpox, diphtheria, diarrhea and enteritis, measles, meningitis, cholera, pneumonia, tuberculosis, typhoid fever, syphilis etc. Today, many of these diseases have effective treatment options and smallpox—once the leading cause of death —has now been globally eradicated. However, the growing resistance to available antibiotics and failure to develop new ones is pointing towards a reversal of the successes of the past century.

## Sepsis Treatment

Sepsis is a common condition characterized by blood poisoning caused by the immune system's dysregulated response to bacterial infections. Though this occurs in extreme cases, any bacterial infection—especially if left untreated—can result in the development of sepsis. The growing number of bacterial infections caused by drug resistant pathogenic bacteria is gravely contributing to the number of people who become ill with sepsis, and this number is only expected to dramatically increase. In 2017, approximately 49 million cases were recorded, and sepsis accounted for almost 20% of all global deaths or 11 million people. Sepsis is largely a result of bacterial infections acquired from healthcare settings, which are often resistant to antibiotics. 1 in 3 patients who are admitted in the hospital for sepsis die. The high mortality rate is due to a lack of accurate early-stage diagnostic methods, treatment options and the rapid deterioration of clinical manifestations, leading to tissue damage, organ failure and death. According to WHO, of the 49 million cases in 2017, over 20 million sepsis cases and 3 million deaths occured in children under five years of age, which is a faint echo of the pre-antibiotic era where the death of infants and children under 5 were widespread.

## Surgery

Surgical site infections account for up to 20% of all healthcare-acquired infections and are caused by bacteria that enter the body through incisions made during surgery. These infections are largely resistant to antibiotics and can result in a longer length of stay in the hospital, readmission or even death. Orthopaedic operations (including joint and hip replacement surgeries), caesarean sections, and oral surgeries are examples of common procedures that are at high risk for causing surgical site infections. In surgical practice, antibacterial agents are used in all three stages: preoperative for prophylaxis, intraoperative to sanitize tools, and postoperative to treat surgical site infections. Antibiotic prophylaxis is the practice of prescribing short-term antibiotics preoperatively to reduce the incidence of surgical site infections. The decision to administer antibiotic prophylaxis is meticulously assessed by weighing the risks and benefits. Evidence supporting routine administration of antibiotic prophylaxis continues to grow, with one study demonstrating a 80% reduction in the absolute risk of surgical wound infection. However, the inappropriate use of antibiotics may lead to resistant infections in the long term. The routine antibiotic prophylactic administration is standard in surgeries involving artificial or foreign body implants, bone grafting, extensive dissection, or those with expected high blood loss. The absence of preoperative antibiotic prescription leads to an increased risk of largely-resistant surgical-site infections, which may result in severe outcomes including death. Furthermore, individuals undergoing complex surgeries, such as organ transplants, receive immunosuppressors which further weaken the immune system's ability to fight infections. Without effective antibiotics to prevent and treat surgical infections, it would be impossible to perform many of these critical, life-saving surgeries. To put this into perspective, over 313 million surgeries occurred globally in 2018, and the growing antibiotic resistance crisis may result in a gravely larger number of annual indirect deaths than the predicted 10 million by 2050.

## Chronic Conditions

Chronic diseases are conditions that last one year or more and require continual medical intervention or limit one's ability to carry out daily activities. They are often characterized by long duration and slow progression. These may include diabetes mellitus, obesity, cardiovascular diseases (such as heart attacks and stroke), chronic respiratory diseases (like chronic obstructive pulmonary disease (COPD) and asthma) etc. The onset of chronic diseases and the medications used to treat them weaken the immune system, thereby reducing the body's ability to fight bacterial infections. Diabetes mellitus is a chronic, metabolic disease that is characterized by elevated levels of blood sugar. A retrospective, large cohort study analyzing a primary care database (representative of the U.K. population) found a significant increase in the risk of developing infections in patients with diabetes mellitus. Crude infection rate is the number of new cases of infection occurring in a specified population per year. The study found the crude rates to be consistently high across 18 different infectious disease categories. According to the WHO, diabetes mellitus affects approximately 422 million people globally, and 1.6 million people die as a direct result each year. Looking at the increasing incidence of obesity in recent decades, emerging data indicates an association between obesity and the incidence of infectious diseases. The WHO defines obesity as abnormal or excessive fat accumulation with a Body Mass Index greater than or equal to 30. Though the underlying mechanism is unknown, this increase in infectious diseases may be due to obesity-related immune system dysregulation, comorbidities such as hypertension and diabetes mellitus associated with obesity, and respiratory dysfunction. With a higher risk of developing infections and an increase in antibiotic resistance, individuals with chronic conditions will be at an enormously higher risk of infection.

## Dialysis for Advanced Kidney Disease

Patients suffering from advanced-stage chronic kidney disease need to undergo dialysis or kidney transplantation, in case of kidney failure. Chronic kidney disease is a long-term condition where the ability of the kidneys to perform their function deteriorates over time, ultimately leading to kidney failure in the end stages. In 2017, the global prevalence of chronic kidney disease was 9.1% or 697.5 million cases. The ineffective diagnostic tools lead to most patients being diagnosed at later stages, leaving dialysis or kidney transplantation as the only treatment options for many. The association of bacterial infections and surgical operations such as kidney transplantation have been previously established. Patients who receive dialysis treatment have a high risk of post-treatment infection, which is the second leading cause of death in dialysis patients. A study published in February 2020 revealed a strong incidence of post-dialysis infection in patients with advanced chronic kidney disease. The findings were consistent with a previous study analyzing the incidence of infectious diseases in 333,453 dialysis patients, where patients were found to have a higher probability of contracting these diseases up to 3 years after the treatment. Each infectious disease event post-dialysis treatment results in worsening nutritional status, readmission and cardiovascular events in these patients. The prevalence of antibiotic-resistant bacterial infections has been found to dramatically increase in the last two decades, with health care settings including outpatient dialysis facilities becoming prominent infection sites. The antibiotic resistant strains known to cause these infections in dialysis patients top the WHO's list of priority pathogens. Antibiotics are vital drugs for these patients and the growing resistance rates will lead to a higher risk of complications from infectious diseases, reduced ability of patients to receive these life-saving dialysis treatments, and increased death rate.

## Cancer Care

Major strides in cancer treatment have researchers and clinicians hopeful of achieving their long-held dream of turning a diagnosis of cancer from a death sentence to a chronic illness. However, the silent pandemic of antibiotic resistance is calling the future of cancer treatment into question. Cancer is a leading cause of death globally, claiming nearly 10 million deaths in 2020. Surgery and radiation therapy served as the gold standard for cancer treatment for decades, however are limited by their ability to only treat malignant cancers locally confined to one organ. With increased understanding of cancer as a systemic disease, chemotherapy and targeted molecular therapy kill cancer cells that have metastasized to distant parts of the body. Immune suppression associated with cancer occurs primarily as a result of reduced white blood cells (also known as leukocytes), which play a key role in the body's defence mechanism. Neutrophils are hematopoietic-derived leukocytes that serve as the first line of defense during inflammation and exogenous infections. They have a well established role in promoting bacterial clearance during infection by being recruited to the site of inflammation, caused by the invading bacteria. In a majority of cancer patients, neutropenia—clinically significant lowered levels of neutrophils — often occurs as a side effect of chemotherapy. Given that leukocytes—along with cancer cells— grow rapidly, they are unfortunately also affected by chemotherapy. As a result, the body's ability to fight infectious diseases becomes compromised. Increased susceptibility to bacterial infections and weak defense mechanisms result in the increased possibility of a cancer patient to have sepsis. Bacterial infections in cancer patients can result in overnight hospitalization, intensive care unit admissions, and even death. In the USA alone, sepsis is responsible for nearly 1 in 10 cancer deaths. Despite aggressive care, cancer patients have a higher hospital mortality rate upon developing sepsis than those who are cancer-free. This is largely because cancer patients are at a high-risk of developing antibiotic resistant infections, given that they frequent healthcare settings. In the absence of effective antibiotics, oncologists may not be able to administer chemotherapy in the future and the therapeutic benefit of the treatment will be greatly reduced.

The use of antibiotics in modern medicine is widespread and their application seems to be further ingrained in the system than what meets the eye. In addition to being used for treating bacterial infections, antibiotics are used in a significant capacity in most clinical practices—from surgery to treating secondary infections. The threat of antibiotic resistance is real and is increasingly threatening the advances made in modern medicine over the last century.

# Chapter 4: Underlying Mechanisms and Causes of Antibiotic Resistance

By: Dr. Austin Mardon & Maryam Oloriegbe

Bacteria can utilize multiple biochemical pathways to evade antimicrobial drugs, making it difficult to target one mechanism and inhibit the resistance of bacteria. Furthermore, many bacteria can use one or more mechanisms of resistance to suppress antibiotic action and survive their effect. There are four common mechanisms in which antibiotic resistance occurs: limiting the uptake of a drug, modifying the drug target, inactivating the antibiotic drug, and actively effluxing the antibiotic out of the bacterial cell.

## Modifying the drug target

Antibiotics target different bacterial cell wall components; however, every one of those targets is modifiable to confer resistance against the drug(s). One of the main targets is the cell wall. Drugs such as vancomycin and daptomycin work by inhibiting cell wall synthesis or depolarizing the cell membrane to disable the entry and exit of molecules in and out of the bacterial cell wall; depolarizing drugs such as daptomycin work in the presence of a positive ion such as calcium or sodium to bind (Reygaert, 2018). However, to confer resistance, a mutation in a gene will cause the charge of the cell wall to switch to positive, repelling the positive charge of the calcium and thus inhibiting daptomycin (Reygaert, 2018).

Bacteria can also gain resistance to drugs that target the ribosome. Ribosomal mutations usually inhibit antibiotics containing aminoglycosides and oxazolidinones. Oxazolidinones are synthetic bacteriostatic antibiotics that target and exert their influence by binding specifically to the A site of the bacterial ribosome, inhibiting protein synthesis by interfering with aminoacyl-RNA positioning (Reygaert, 2018). Linezolid, a specific type of oxazolidinone, is the most widely used antibiotic of the drug type. Resistance to it typically occurs with mutations in the genes encoding the domain V of 23S rRNA in the 50S subunit (Reygaert, 2018). Interestingly, bacteria carry multiple copies of the 23S rRNA gene; therefore, mutation accumulation must occur through most if not all alleles to yield a bacterial resistant phenotype and decrease linezolid's affinity for the bacterial ribosome (Munita & Arias, 2016).

With gram-positive bacteria, macrolide and streptogramins containing drugs are inhibited by ribosomal subunit methylation. Ribosome protection is another mechanism of resistance in which ribosomal protection proteins (RPPs) dislodge antibiotics such as tetracycline from the bacterial ribosome binding sites (Reygaert, 2018).

Some antibacterial drugs such as fluoroquinolones target

components of nucleic acid synthesis, including DNA topoisomerase in gram-positive bacteria and DNA gyrase (a type of topoisomerase) in gram-negative bacteria (Reygaert, 2018). Resistance occurs through mutation of gyrase and topoisomerase, which hinders the ability of the drug to bind to both structures to inhibit them, rendering nucleic acid synthesis successful in bacteria (Reygaert, 2018).

The last method of modification of the drug target is modifying the metabolic pathway in which drugs that attempt to hinder a step in a specific pathway in bacteria are inhibited through a mutation in one or more of the enzymes involved in the metabolic pathway. In the case of folic acid synthesis, which many bacteria depend on for their growth and survival, antimicrobials will bind to the active site of the dihydropteroate synthase and dihydrofolate reductase (DHPS and DHFR) enzymes through competitive inhibition, for which they can do because the drug contains a structural analog that is similar in shape and size to the substrate in the pathway (eg. the drug-containing sulfonamide has a similar structure to p-aminobenzoic acid (PABA), the natural substrate that binds to DHPS; trimethoprim has a similar structure to dihydrofolate (DHF), the natural substrate that binds to DHFR) (Munita & Arias, 2016). However, to confer resistance, DHPS and DHPR will mutate a gene in or near their active site to prevent the binding and competitive inhibition of sulfonamide and trimethoprim while simultaneously allowing PABA and DHF, the natural substrates, to bind (Munita & Arias, 2016).

## Inactivation of the drug

One of the most successful ways bacteria cope and survive with the presence of antibiotics is modifying the drug to either chemically alter or destroy the drug, rendering it unable to bind to the target.

A well-known mechanism that both gram-positive and gram-negative bacteria utilize to chemical alter the antibiotic (typically ones that inhibit protein synthesis at the ribosomal level) is the production of specific enzymes that induce enzyme modification. Such modifications include acetylation, phosphorylation, and adenylation. These biochemical reactions decrease the antibiotic's ability to bind to the target (Munita & Arias, 2016).

One example of resistance via modification of the drug is the production of the aminoglycoside modifying enzymes (AME), responsible for modifying the hydroxyl or amino groups of the aminoglycoside compound in antibiotics (Munita & Arias, 2016). Additionally, phosphorylation and adenylation-type reactions are known to modify aminoglycosides primarily (Reygaert, 2018).

Another classic example is the modification of the antibiotic chloramphenicol, which inhibits protein synthesis by interacting with the T site on the 50S ribosome (Munita & Arias, 2016). Bacterial acetyltransferase enzymes, known as chloramphenicol acetyltransferases (CATs), are responsible for their modification in both gram-positive and gram-negative bacteria and are further classified into Types A and B; the former resulting in high-level resistance and the latter resulting in a much lower level of resistance (Munita & Arias, 2016).

Finally, the most common and widely used antibiotic in the market, the β-lactam drug, consists of a core and a specific four-sided ring, depending on the class of β-lactam (Class A, B, C, D). These drugs can be inactivated either by destroying the amide bond in the ring (via the β-lactamase enzymes in the bacteria) or modifying the structure of the β-lactam so that it can not bind to penicillin-binding proteins (PBP), rendering it inactive against bacteria (C Reygaert, 2018.

## Drug Efflux

Bacteria possess chromosomal genes that encode efflux pumps. These efflux pumps are responsible for removing unwanted toxic substances from the bacteria. Many bacteria have pumps, known as multi-drug resistant (MDR) pumps, that efflux many substances that allow them to gain multi-drug resistance against many different antibiotics. Efflux pumps can be characterized in gram-positive and gram-negative bacteria as substrate-specific or have broad state specificity, such as in MDR bacteria (Munita & Arias, 2016). There are five prominent families of efflux pumps, of which many bacteria can possess multiple families depending on their resistance to certain antibiotics. They include the ATP-binding cassette (ABC) family, the multidrug and toxic compound extrusion (MATE) family, the small multidrug resistance (SMR) family, the major facilitator superfamily (MFS), and the resistance-nodulation-cell division (RND) family (Reygaert, 2018). Due to the wide range of efflux pumps, many antibiotics, many of which target specific components of the bacterial cell, such as protein synthesis inhibitors, fluoroquinolones, β-lactams, carbapenems and polymyxins, can be effluxed from the bacteria and rendered ineffective against a specific bacterium or even a species of bacteria (Reygaert, 2018).

Regarding the families of efflux pumps, each family "differ in terms of structural conformation, energy source, range of substrates they are able to extrude and in the type of bacterial organisms in which they are distributed" (Munita & Arias, 2016). The ABC transporter family possesses uptake (taking substances into the bacterial cell) and efflux transport systems. Using the energy of ATP hydrolysis, they transport amino acids, ions, drugs, polysaccharides and sugars. Because of their specificity for specific substrates, they are found in very few clinically significant bacteria (Reygaert, 2018). However, the most notable ABC pump is in the *Vibrio cholerae* bacteria and can transport fluoroquinolones and tetracycline (Reygaert, 2018).

The SMR transporter family, which utilizes energy by the proton-motive force, are hydrophobic proteins that extrude mainly lipophilic cations, making the substrate range extremely narrow. Unlike ABC transporters, SMR transporters do not uptake substances, only effluxing β-lactams and some aminoglycosides. They are also typically seen in bacteria such as *Staphylococcus epidermidis* and Escherichia coli (Reygaert, 2018).

The MATE transporter family uses a sodium ion gradient as its energy source. MATE pumps tend to efflux cationic dyes and fluoroquinolone drugs, with a few pumps shown to efflux aminoglycosides. While very few types of MATE pumps have been categorized, most have been found in gram-negative bacteria. Some notable examples of bacteria possessing MATE pumps include *Vibrio parahaemolyticus* with the NorM pump from its chromosomal DNA, *Neisseria gonorrhoeae,* and *Neisseria meningitidis*, which have also been shown to possess the NorM pump (Reygaert, 2018).

The RND transporter family utilizes a substrate/H+ antiport mechanism and is found in many gram-negative bacteria. Along with the efflux of multiple antibiotics (multi-drug transporters), they are also involved in removing detergents, dyes, heavy metals, solvents, and other substrates. Most RND pumps are capable of transporting a wide range of antibiotics independent of the type or class of drug. The most widely studied RND pump is the AcrAB-TolC pump in *Escherichia coli* and confers resistance to penicillins, chloramphenicol, macrolides, fluoroquinolones, and tetracycline (Reygaert, 2018).

The final efflux pump family, the MFS transporters, catalyze transport via a solute/sodium symport, solute/proton symport or solute/proton antiport. They transport anions, drugs, metabolites, and sugars. Generally, MFS pumps have a wide range of substrate diversity but have substrate specificity as individual pumps. *Acinetobacter baumannii* has separate MFS pumps for the erythromycin and chloramphenicol antibiotics, *E. coli* has separate MFS pumps for macrolides, fluoroquinolones, and trimethoprim (Reygaert, 2018). In addition, over 50% of *E. coli* pumps are MFS transporters and are typically encoded from bacterial chromosomes.

One of the most notable examples of efflux pumps is the Tet

efflux pump, under the MFS family. These are responsible for extruding tetracycline antibiotics to confer resistance to the bacteria. About 20 tet genes have been examined and described, with a majority of them being found in gram-negative bacteria and only the Tet(K) and Tet(L) genes being among the exceptions found in gram-positive bacteria. As there are different types of tetracycline antibiotics, such as minocycline, doxycycline, and tigecycline, many pumps can affect some variants of the tetracycline antibiotics but not others. Some efflux pumps can even extrude the antibiotics but will not decrease the overall susceptibility of the bacteria to the drug due to the inability to use the compounds as substrates (Munita & Arias, 2016; as cited in K Poole, 2005 and MC Roberts, 2005).

Macrolide antibiotics are also affected by bacteria's efflux mechanism through the *mef* genes that encode the mefA and mefE efflux pumps resulting in macrolide resistance. Mef pumps are typically found in *Streptococcus pyogenes* and *Staphylococcus pneumoniae,* in addition to other streptococci and gram-positive bacteria. Moreover, cross-resistance was not examined across streptogramins and lincosamides; although the antibiotics are effective against gram-positive bacteria like macrolides, bacteria typically can not confer resistance against them (Munita & Arias, 2016).

## Limiting Drug Uptake

While many antibiotics are designed to target the cell wall and other extracellular components, some are designed to target intracellular components such as the ribosomes to target bacterial protein synthesis. To do this, the antimicrobial must penetrate the outer and inner walls of the cytoplasmic membrane to initiate its effect on the bacteria. However, bacteria have developed mechanisms to gain resistance against that effect by limiting the drug uptake or decreasing the permeability of the outer cell and inner cytoplasmic membrane, so penetration is not possible. This is especially important in gram-negative bacteria when conferring resistance against hydrophilic molecules. They have a thinner peptidoglycan layer compared to the thicker layer found in gram-positive bacteria. Furthermore, gram-negative bacteria have a lipopolysaccharide (LPS) layer, which further acts as a barrier against specific hydrophilic antimicrobials, such as β-lactams, tetracyclines and some fluoroquinolones, which can not penetrate a hydrophobic membrane.

The specific mechanism involved in limiting drug uptake has to do with the number or differential expression of porins, beta-barrel proteins that cross the cell membrane and act as a pore for usually small hydrophilic molecules to passively diffuse through (Munita & Arias, 2016). Porins can be classified according to their structure, selectivity, and how their expression is regulated. *E. coli* has some of the most classic examples of porins with the three major proteins produced as OmpF, OmpC, and PhoE (Munita & Arias, 2016). They, and all other porin proteins, alter the permeability of the cell membrane in three ways: shifting the type of porin being expressed, changing the level of porin expression (reducing the number), or impairing the function of the porin so nothing can pass through (Munita & Arias, 2016). Because some porins are still being expressed, this usually results in low-level resistance against antibiotics; thus, this mechanism is typically associated with other mechanisms of resistance, such as increasing the expression of efflux pumps (Munita & Arias, 2016 as cited in Nikaido, 2003decrease).

Another interesting example was found in an experiment studying *Klebsiella pneumoniae*, a gram-negative bacteria (Munita & Arias, 2016). Scientists obtained clinical isolates, treated them with antimicrobial therapy, and compared them before and after treatment (Munita & Arias, 2016). They found that the post-therapy isolates had shifted porin expression from OmpK35 to OmpK36, which exhibited a decrease in channel size. The smaller channel directly correlates with a decrease in susceptibility to β-lactam antibiotics (Munita & Arias, 2016). Similar examples were seen in *Enterobacter cloacae, Salmonella spp., Neisseria gonorrhoeae,* and *A. baumannii,* all of which are species of clinical importance (Munita & Arias, 2016).

Collectively, bacteria possess an impressive ability to form a biofilm through various microorganisms in a bacterial community. Biofilms protect the bacteria from an attack by the immune system and provide protection against antibiotics (Reygaert, 2018). It contains polysaccharides, proteins, and DNA from the bacteria community to form a thick and sticky layer, making it difficult for immune cells and antibiotics to reach and penetrate the bacteria. As a result, higher concentrations of antimicrobial drugs are needed to overcome the sticky matrix. However, drugs that target the growth and division of bacteria would be rendered ineffective as bacterial cells in the biofilm tend to be sessile or undergo slow division and have a slow metabolism rate (Reygaert, 2018). A crucial and yet terrifying observation is that horizontal gene transfer can occur between bacterial cells within the biofilm due to their proximity; therefore, making the sharing of antibiotic resistance genes potentially easier (Reygaert, 2018).

## *Staphylococcus aureus*: A bacteria of many mechanisms

Considered to be one of the most versatile microorganisms to date, *S. aureus* is the most widespread organism and one of the leading causes of disease worldwide. Many antibiotics have been created to target different components of the gram-positive bacteria; however, within a few years of discovery, *S. aureus* began to show resistance, resulting in almost all strains of the bacteria becoming resistant and being extremely difficult to treat. The first antibiotic to be used against *S. aureus* was penicillin, discovered in the 1940s (Reygaert, 2013). After gaining resistance against the drug, researchers sought to find different variations and modifications of penicillin that would target different areas of the bacteria (Reygaert, 2013). Eventually, other β-lactam compounds were discovered and utilized, although they had weak antimicrobial activity (Reygaert, 2013). However, it was found that they were capable of inhibiting β-lactamase enzymes, proteins produced by *S. aureus* to fight the β-lactam compounds, specifically hydrolyzing the peptide bond in the β-lactam ring to inactivate it. Researchers developed ampicillin, oxacillin, and methicillin to prevent the β-lactams attack and instead bind to PBPs without any unwarranted intervention from the bacteria. However, *S. aureus* utilized another mechanism, modification of the drug target, to evade the modified penicillin antibiotics. The *mecA* gene expresses PBP2a, a new PBP with a lower affinity to methicillin, rendering it ineffective in binding (Reygaert, 2013). Vancomycin, an antibacterial drug that targets cell wall synthesis, had promising results due to the small number of reports of resistance; nevertheless, the possibility of resistance becoming an issue is increasing over the years. *S. aureus* can gain resistance against vancomycin in two ways. Vancomycin-intermediate *S. aureus* (VISA) resistance occurs through the thickening of the cell wall, so vancomycin can not penetrate and enter the cell. Vancomycin-resistant *S. aureus* (VRSA) acquires the *vanA* gene and is mediated through modification of the peptidoglycan precursors, decreasing binding affinity for vancomycin (Reygaert, 2013). Both mechanisms of vancomycin resistance utilize modification of the drug target to inhibit the antibiotic from binding to the bacterial cell wall.

## Conclusion

Understanding antibiotic resistance mechanisms help researchers develop antibiotics that target different bacterial components while evading other bacteria's defence systems. Despite this, bacteria can evolve to gain additional, more complex mechanisms that make it difficult for antibiotics to target their respective components. As a result, antibiotic resistance is rapidly becoming one of the greatest public threats of the 21st century and is only set to make bacterial infections ever more untreatable.

# Chapter 5: Therapeutic Challenges in the Era of Antibiotic Resistance

By: Dr. Austin Mardon & Gurman Barara

## Introduction

Antibiotic resistance is an enormous concern in the field of medicine. This ongoing crisis has led to many challenges when treating infection such as higher medical costs, increased hospital stays, and higher mortality due to pathogenic bacteria (World Health Organization, 2020). Antibiotic resistant bacteria, when present in the human body, can be quite difficult to treat as the standard course of antibiotics will be ineffective. A lot of research is dedicated to determining effective treatment for resistant bacteria. Treatment options include the use of multiple drugs simultaneously, the development of new antibiotics, and the use of alternative antibiotics with the same underlying mechanisms (Lee, 2008). Although the treatment options seem to be effective in treating bacterial infections, there are quite a lot of challenges presented with treating antibiotic resistant bacteria. The misuse of antibiotics contributes to the development of antibiotic resistance as well (Ventola, 2015).

## Misuse of Antibiotics

The misuse of antibiotics strongly contributes to antibiotic resistance and therapeutic challenges associated with this phenomenon. This means that they are prescribed by a physician without truly knowing the cause of infection (Ventola, 2015). This is also referred to as "blinded use". In an ideal situation, the physician would first take a sample of the infection to identify the pathogen and then prescribe a drug after the pathogen has been identified. Blinded use of antibiotics may sometimes be inappropriate and can lead to bacteria developing resistance. Viral infections can sometimes be mistaken for bacterial infections as well. Antibiotics would be ineffective against viral infections because their mechanisms of actions are selective for bacteria only. Having said that, it would be inappropriate to prescribe antibiotics to a patient with a viral infection. This does, however, happen in reality and is something that physicians and patients must be wary of.

Antibiotics are also used in livestock. Although many countries have banned or limited the use of antibiotics in raising livestock (including Canada), some countries continue to use antibiotics when raising animals. The use of antibiotics in livestock is to promote growth and prevent bacterial infection (Ventola, 2015). Antibiotics are primarily used by farmers because it helps animals to gain weight faster, thus producing more meat in a shorter amount of time. Antibiotics in animal feed may be a cost-effective method for generating more meat products; however, it can lead to antibiotic resistance amongst livestock and humans. If antibiotics are used in animals for growth, bacteria may develop resistance and cause infection that may be difficult to treat in animals. This can take a deadly toll on livestock and the meat industry. Not to mention, the bacteria may be able to transmit to humans and cause infection as well (Ventola, 2015).

Another misuse of antibiotics that can lead to resistance is when patients do not complete the full course of the drug (Ventola, 2015). For instance, a patient diagnosed with pulmonary tuberculosis caused by the bacteria *Mycobacterium tuberculosis* would generally be prescribed the antibiotics isoniazid and rifampicin. The course of these drugs is usually for a period of 6 months (National Health Service, 2019). A patient may begin to exhibit fewer symptoms associated with tuberculosis after the first 2-3 months and then may decide to stop using the antibiotics because they are feeling better. However, not all the pathogenic bacteria in the body may have been eradicated and can continue to replicate and cause infection in the absence of these antibiotics. The pathogen may then develop mechanisms to be resistant to isoniazid and rifampicin due to selective pressures. In this situation, the pathogen would become resistant to more than one drug and may be very difficult to treat.

## Multidrug Therapy

When one type of antibiotic is prescribed to a patient, the pathogenic bacteria may be resistant and thus, the antibiotic will be inefficient at treating the infection. A possible treatment to antibiotic resistant bacteria is the use of multidrug therapy. In this situation, a mixture of antibiotic drugs are prescribed to the patient with the aim to eradicate the bacterial infection. When prescribing a mixture of drugs, it is important to ensure that there are no adverse reactions and drug-drug interactions between the prescribed drugs.

Multidrug therapy is considered as an option because when a mixture of drugs are given at one time, the chances of bacterial pathogens developing resistance to the drugs is low. In other words, bacteria are more likely to develop resistance to one type of antibiotic rather than a mixture of several drugs. It must be taken into consideration that bacteria can, although very unlikely, develop resistance to multiple drugs. The selection pressures of combination drug therapy can lead to an overall rise in resistance amongst bacteria. This type of antibiotic resistance is called multidrug resistance. If bacteria develop multidrug resistance,the infection can be life threatening and treatment is often very difficult (Nikaido, 2009).

Several studies have shown that the use of multidrug therapy is more effective at treating infection than single drug therapy. Overall, mortality rates in patients receiving multidrug therapy was lower than patients receiving single antibiotic drug therapy (Schmid et al., 2019).

Although combination drug therapy is seen as a treatment option to antibiotic resistance, there are several disadvantages that must be considered as well. Multidrug therapy is often more expensive and results in higher medical costs. Moreover, this form of therapy can lead to adverse reactions and can potentially lead to nephrotoxicity (kidney toxicity). If bacteria develop resistance to multidrug therapy, then selection pressures will favour bacteria that are resistant to several antibiotics. Although this is highly unlikely, it is still possible and can lead to the development of multidrug resistant bacterial infections, which can be difficult to treat (Nikaido, 2009). Lastly, the simultaneous use of multiple antibiotics has the possibility to eradicate the human flora more quickly than single drug therapy (bacteria that are non-pathogenic and reside in humans). This can lead to infection by bacteria called opportunistic pathogens.

## Opportunistic Pathogens

There are a variety of bacterial species which live in or on the human body. These bacteria can be referred to as "normal bacterial flora". It must be mentioned that not all bacteria are pathogenic (cause infection). These bacteria, which comprise the human flora, are also called the "good bacteria" and have a symbiotic relationship with humans. Specifically, the type of relationship between humans and the normal flora is mutualistic —both the bacteria and host benefit from one another. For example, the normal human flora carry out several functions such as assisting in digestion and absorption of nutrients, synthesis of vitamin K, protection against pathogens etc (National Institutes of Health, 2012). This is beneficial to human hosts. On the other hand, the bacteria are benefitted as they can thrive in the human body and are provided with nutrients.

A challenge with antibiotic therapy is that pathogens and normal bacterial flora in the gut are eliminated. This in turn, can lead to diarrhea, nausea, compromised breakdown of food etc.

Moreover, the normal human flora consists of bacteria which prevent the colonization of pathogens by competing for nutrients. When antibiotics eradicate the normal gut bacteria, or good bacteria, this can allow pathogenic bacteria to thrive as there is no competition for nutrients. These infectious bacteria that thrive under these conditions are called opportunistic pathogens. An example of an opportunistic pathogen is the bacteria *Clostridium difficile*.

*C. difficile* is a pathogen that can exist in the large intestine and is often found in hospitals and nursing homes. *C. difficile* can lead to pseudomembranous colitis—swelling or inflammation of the large intestine—and the biggest risk factor for this condition is previous antibiotic treatment. When patients receive antibiotics to treat infection, the normal microbiota in the intestine is also killed. This allows opportunistic pathogens such as *C. difficile* to thrive in an environment where "good bacteria" are absent and produce toxins that can cause fever, diarrhea, abdominal pain, swelling of the large intestine and dehydration (Liubakka and Vaughn, 2016).

The antibiotic vancomycin can be used to treat *C. difficile* infections. However, treatment of *C. difficile* through the use of antibiotics can sometimes be quite ineffective; the use of antibiotics is what allowed this opportunistic pathogen to cause infection in the first place. Rather, *C. difficile* is effectively treated by reintroducing normal human flora into the gut. This is performed through a fecal-oral transplant, also called bacteriotherapy. Bacteria from fecal matter of another individual is placed into the gut of the infected patient (Liubakka and

Vaughn, 2016). As counterintuitive as it seems, this method of treatment has been shown to be efficient in the treatment of infection. The fact that restoring the normal bacterial flora in the gut can treat infections by opportunistic pathogens such as *C. difficile*, shows the importance of the human gut bacteria and highlights the symbiotic relationship between humans and the human microbiome.

Although antibiotics have therapeutic uses because they can eliminate bacterial pathogens, they can also eradicate the normal bacterial flora in humans. This can be quite fatal in that it can lead to compromised breakdown and digestion of food and the potential for opportunistic pathogens to cause infection. This is why it is important to administer a correct dose of antibiotics: a dose high enough to sufficiently kill bacterial pathogens but not too high as to eliminate bacteria which make up the human flora. Another area of research in antibiotic therapy would be to develop drugs which target pathogenic bacteria only, rather than eliminating the normal bacterial flora in humans as well.

## Use of Alternative Antibiotics

Similar to *C. difficile*, another opportunistic pathogen is the bacteria *Staphylococcus aureus*. *S. aureus* is a pathogenic bacteria that can cause abscesses (boils), sinusitis, or more serious infections such as pneumonia or sepsis. *S. aureus* is commonly found in the human bacterial flora in 30% of the population (Tong et al., 2015). These carriers are usually healthy and asymptomatic.

The bacteria usually colonizes on the skin and mucosal

membranes and can be transmitted from direct skin to skin contact. *S. aureus* can cause infection when it enters open wounds or binds proteins on cell surface receptors which can allow widespread colonization (Choo and Chambers, 2016). Infection by *S. aureus* often leads to the development of skin lesions known as abscesses. These abscesses are most frequent on the skin but can occur in organs as well, which can be a lot more serious. Abscesses are a collection of dead neutrophils (white blood cells) which form pus due to infection. Treatment is required to heal these abscesses and typically includes draining the pus and antibiotic therapy.

Another infection caused by *S. aureus* is osteomyelitis—the infection of the bone or bone marrow. This usually occurs when the *S. aureus* pathogen contaminates the bones during an injury, orthopaedic surgery or the infection spreads to the bone by other methods (Reizner et al., 2014). Treatment involves surgical removal of damaged tissue and the administration of antibiotics intravenously.

As mentioned above, the infections caused by *S. aureus* require antibiotic therapy for treatment. Otherwise, the consequences can be quite lethal. The two types of infections mentioned— abscesses and osteomyelitis—often occur in a hospital environment. Having said that, *S. aureus* strains in hospitals have been known to have evolved and become resistant to the antibiotic methicillin. As such, these are called hospital-associated methicillin resistant *Staphylococcus aureus* (MRSA). *S. aureus* strains that have evolved resistance to methicillin are quite dangerous because methicillin is usually the standard treatment for *S. aureus* infections. Having said that, when methicillin is prescribed to a patient infected with MRSA, the good bacteria in the body will be killed by the antibiotics yet, the *S. aureus* will continue to thrive in the absence of the human flora. This is quite problematic and can cause severe infections and health problems.

To overcome infections by MRSA, the antibiotic vancomycin can be prescribed. Although some resistance to vancomycin has also been reported, it is still an effective therapy to treat infections caused by strains of *S. aureus* resistant to methicillin (Choo and Chambers, 2016). A downside of using vancomycin, however, is that it can lead to nephrotoxicity (kidney damage). With that being said, long term use of vancomycin is not ideal.

The use of alternative antibiotics to treat antibiotic resistant strains of bacteria can be an effective therapy. However, as it can be seen, the use of alternative drugs may have certain adverse effects or may not be as well tolerated amongst patients. This is another barrier in antibiotic therapy that must be overcome.

## Allergic Reactions

Allergic reactions to antibiotics is a significant concern for some patients. Some common signs of allergic reactions include hives, swelling, coughing and difficulty breathing, itchy skin etc. About 1 in 15 people experience allergic reactions to antibiotics and the most common allergic reaction is caused by the antibiotic penicillin (National Health Service, 2021). Penicillins are effective against gram positive bacteria, however, patients with a penicillin allergy should avoid the use of penicillin and drugs that fall within the same class or have similar mechanisms. For example, cephalosporins are another class of antibiotics with similar mechanisms of action as the penicillins. These drugs can act as a suitable alternative for penicillins and can be used safely by patients with a penicillin allergy (Pichichero, 2006).

If patients are experiencing an allergic reaction to antibiotics, then the drug should be stopped immediately and an antihistamine and epinephrine can be administered accordingly.

## Development of New Antibiotic Drugs

Antibiotic resistance is developed by bacteria to drugs that were once effective. Once bacteria develop resistance to one type of drug, a new drug can be developed to eradicate the bacteria. However, this is not an ideal and permanent solution because bacteria will continue to evolve resistance mechanisms and selection will favour antibiotic resistant strains.

Pharmaceutical companies are not as invested in antibiotics as other drugs because antibiotic resistance is inevitable (Boseley, 2020). Bacteria and humans are at a constant evolutionary arms race and bacterial pathogens are constantly evolving and developing new mechanisms to thrive and cause infection in human hosts (even in the presence of antibiotics). The introduction of new drugs to the market is a time consuming and expensive process. There are several steps that must be met for the approval of drugs such as preclinical testing, and multiple phases of clinical trials. This process can take up to 10-15 years and monetary investments of hundreds of millions of dollars

(Wellcome, 2020).

*Neisseria gonorrhoeae* bacterial cultures are evolving to develop resistance to several classes of antibiotics (Public Health Agency of Canada, 2016). In general, these bacteria have developed the most resistance to tetracycline antibiotics over a 10 year period from 2004 to 2014. About 50% of bacterial cultures that exhibited tetracycline resistance were able to be isolated in 2014.

As mentioned earlier, bacteria are constantly evolving and developing mechanisms for antibiotic resistance. Although newly developed antibiotics may be successful at first to eradicate previously resistant bacteria, bacteria will eventually develop mechanisms for resistance to new drugs. An example of this can be seen in *N. gonorrhoeae* cultures—where there is an upward trend in cultures that develop resistance to antibiotics over time (Public Health Agency of Canada, 2016). Not to mention, newly developed antibiotics are not sold in large volumes and are often used as a last resort for dangerous pathogens (Wellcome, 2020). This is done to limit overuse and the development of antibiotic resistance. Antibiotics are also relatively cheap drugs, meaning there is not a high profit margin for pharmaceutical companies. From a business standpoint, the return of investment on antibiotics is quite low and not very profitable.

As such, the high investment on developing new drugs but the low return has caused a lot of pharmaceutical companies to withdraw from antibiotic development as it is simply not profitable. The development of new antibiotic drugs is very limited and is not sufficient to combat the emerging antibiotic resistance crisis (Wellcome, 2020).

## Conclusion

The phenomenon of antibiotic resistance is an emerging global crisis in the treatment of bacterial infection. Bacteria are constantly evolving to develop mechanisms to evade the bactericidal and bacteriostatic effects of antibiotics. The development of new antibiotics, the use of alternative drugs and using multidrug therapy are all limited solutions to combat bacterial antibiotic resistance. The misuse of antibiotics should be minimized to allow for efficient treatment of bacterial infections.

# Chapter 6: Nanotechnology as a Therapeutic Tool

By: Dr. Austin Mardon & Tolu Atama

## Background

The emergence of nanotechnology to treat antimicrobial resistance (AMR) occurred because in the past few decades antimicrobial resistance became increasingly difficult to curb. Antimicrobial resistance is a condition that transcends race, gender or nationality – simply put it can affect anyone and is a major threat to healthcare globally. Although, it may occur naturally, improper use of antibiotics increases susceptibility. Conditions such as pneumonia, gonorrhea and tuberculosis have become increasingly difficult to treat as a result of antibiotic resistance (WHO, 2020).

## Epidemiology

Antimicrobial resistance microbes affected a vast number of people in North America and led to increased mortality. The rate of resistance for infections acquired in the hospital and the community is high. Certain bacteria are predominantly more resistant to their associated drugs than others. For example, staphylococcus aureus is second to E-coli and is recorded as one of the most persistent bacteria that resist antibiotics (Akova, 2016). It is resistant to sulfonamide, penicillin, methicillin and vancomycin. More than 50% of staphylococcus aureus types found in hospital-acquired infections are resistant to methicillin and many other antibiotics. The staphylococcus aureus types have caused a longer duration in the hospital, increased treatment dosage and death (Pelgrift and Friedman, 2013).

## Mechanism of Action

To appreciate how nanotechnology curbs antimicrobial resistance, the mechanism by which microbes become resistant to drugs should be understood. There are two main strategies used by the bacteria to resist antibiotics – 1. prevent the antibiotics from reaching the target 2. modify or bypass the target (ReAct, 2021).

### *The process of Preventing the Antibiotics from Reaching the Target*

- *Use of efflux pump:* Microbes remove the antibiotics by a self-pump action. Bacteria produce pumps within their cell membrane which can carry different substances out of the bacteria including antibiotics (CDC, 2020; ReAct, 2021). The pumping lowers the potency of the drug and in some instances increases the resistance depending on the type of pump produced (ReAct, 2021). An example is the ca bacteria which resists antibiotic drugs such as fluoroquinolones beta-lactams, chloramphenicol, and trimethoprim (CDC, 2021).

- *Inhibition of Cell Wall Synthesis:* Some bacteria have no cell wall or can conceal their cell wall; if the drug has a cell wall targeting mechanism of action, it would not affect the bacteria since it has no target (cell wall) to act upon. The former is intrinsic resistance because it has no cell wall and the latter extrinsic because the cell wall is hidden. (ReAct, 2021).
- *Decrease cell membrane permeability:* Some bacteria can restrict access to their cell membrane by changing the composition of the membrane limiting entry into its cell (ReAct, 2021). For example, Gram-negative bacteria can do this because they have a selective membrane that protects them from antibiotic actions (CDC, 2021).
- *Modify/change the antibiotic composition:* Enzymes are also produced to modify the antibiotic composition such that a different chemical substance is added. This makes it impossible for the antibiotic to bind to the bacteria's active site. (ReAct, 2021)
- *Destroying the antibiotic before its action:* Some bacteria can destroy the antibiotics before its action. They release enzymes that inactivate the antibiotics. An example of this is the use of β-lactamase to destroy penicillin, rendering it inactive (ReAct, 2021).
- Also, the enzyme carbapenemase is produced by *Klebsiella pneumoniae* bacteria which destroys

carbapenem drugs and other associated drugs (CDC, 2021).

## The Process of Modifying or By-passing the Target

- *Bypassing the effects of the target of the antibiotic:* Some bacteria produce new cellular protein synthesis that can be used instead of the target. They mimic the target but are not affected by the antibiotic's action. This process allows the actual target to bypass the antibiotics and the bacteria remain untreated. For example, Staphylococcus aureus bacteria resists the action of β-lactam antibiotics using this mechanism of action. This action also produces resistance to penicillin. Methicillin-resistant Staphylococcus aureus - MRSA operates on this type of resistance and mechanism of action (ReAct, 2021). The effect of the drug trimethoprim can also be bypassed using this process (CDC, 2021).
- *Modify the targets for the antibiotics:* The structure of the target in the bacteria is changed preventing the antibiotic from associating with the target. Also, because some drugs are designed to attack a particular part of the bacteria, changes in the structure or shape of the bacteria DNA occur and the drug no longer fits into the shape thus is not able to perform its action. An example of this can be illustrated when Escherichia coli bacteria with the mcr-1 gene adds a substance to the

membrane of its cell wall hence the drug colistin is unable to fasten itself to the cell wall. Thus, the antibiotics cannot perform the required action.

The aforementioned points highlight the need for corrective action. The healthcare burden – resources, cost as well as the increased mortality rate call for a solution. Thus, a solution to alleviate the problem was proposed – nanotechnology.

## Nanotechnology, nanomaterials and nanoparticles

Nanotechnology, defined by the National Nanotechnology Initiative (2021), is the "understanding and control of matter at the nanoscale, at dimensions between approximately 1 and 100 nanometers. Nanotechnology exists in a cross-section between engineering, science and technology, and generally encompasses applications from imaging, materials, measuring, and manipulation of matter at this size and scale."

Also, according to Raj et al (2005) Nanotechnology is the design, characterization, production, and application of structures, devices, and systems by controlled manipulation of size and shape at the nanometer scale (atomic, molecular, and macromolecular scale) that produces structures, devices, and systems with at least one novel/superior characteristic or property.

Nanotechnology, at the nanoscale, produces different types of material, one of which is Nanoparticles (NP). The shape may have varying dimensions and the size of the particle is very tiny.

These unique properties especially the size can affect the physical and chemical characteristics of a substance (Khan et al, 2019).

These attributes of nanotechnology, particularly, its nanoparticle is implicated in its medical application and use to combat antibiotic resistance.

Nanoparticles have been classified in different ways such as organic and inorganic (Eleraky et al, 2019; Natan et al, 2017); metal-based and non-metal based (Natan et al, 2017) nano-carriers (those that transport the antimicrobial portion) and nano-agents (those with intrinsic antibacterial properties) (Natan et al, 2017). Some examples of nanoparticles used to combat antimicrobial resistance processes are liposomes, chitosan, nitric oxide, silver, magnesium, zinc oxide and copper nanoparticles (Eleraky et al, 2019; Munir et al, 2020; Pelgrift and Friedman, 2013).

## Nanotechnology as a therapeutic tool and its role in Antimicrobial Resistance

The increase in antimicrobial resistance is repeatedly attributed to Biofilm and Swarming (Donlan, 2001). Biofilm gives bacteria organisms the ability to tolerate more than one antibiotic drug at an elevated degree. This gives room for repeated infections that are hard to treat. Biofilm is formed when "microorganisms irreversibly attach to and grow on a surface and produce extracellular polymers that facilitate attachment and matrix formation, resulting in an alteration in the phenotype of the organisms with respect to growth rate and gene transcription" (Donlan, 2001). Examples of bacteria that form biofilm are Staphylococcus aureus and Pseudomonas Aeruginosa. Biofilm formations are implicated in a lot of infections such as lung infections and gingivitis, Otitis media and infections related to medical devices (Pelgrift and Friedman, 2013). Swarming is a process where swarm cells are produced within the bacteria causing it to have a high tolerance to antibiotics and evade treatment from multiple antibiotic drugs (Pelgrift and Friedman, 2013).

Nanotechnology is a proven way to combat multiple drug-resistant bacteria. Its role is to fight these bacteria using different types of nanoparticles and mechanisms of actions. Therapeutically, nanotechnology can be used to increase drug dosage by acting primarily at the site of infection thus reducing adverse effects of drugs on patients. Further, it acts by disrupting the mechanism by which bacteria become resistant including biofilm formation, swarming, decrease membrane permeability and an increase in efflux pump out of the antibiotic drug from the membrane of the bacteria (Pelgrift and Friedman, 2013).

## Mechanism of Action of Nanotechnology in Antimicrobial Resistance Prevention

## 1. Nanoparticles with Multiple Combating Tools

Some nanoparticles operate using a method of prevention where more than one mechanism of action is utilized at the same time to fight the bacteria – this process makes the bacteria's mechanism of resistance less likely to work and in turn improve the efficacy of treatment. The following types of nanoparticles utilize this method (Pelgrift and Friedman, 2013).

- *Nitric oxide-releasing nanoparticles (NO-Nps):* NO NP decrease bacteria activity by using multiple antimicrobial activities at the same time to combat the bacteria. This antimicrobial activity happens when NO from the nanoparticles reacts with superoxide (O2-) which forms RNOS reactive nitroxide intermediate.

  At a Nitric oxide level that is above 1mM RNOS effectively activates antibiotic activity via several methods: 1. The reaction of RNOS bacterial protein and amino acid residue. 2. RNOS can damage the DNA structure of the bacteria directly by removal of the amine group and prevent the enzymatic DNA repair actions from occurring. 3. RNOS reacts with the protein prosthetic group and at an elevated amount it binds to the Fe2 which decreases the protein contained in the bacteria thus lowering their activity. 4. RNOS prevents microbial respiration at the cellular level by rendering the zinc metalloproteins contained in some bacteria inactive. 5. In humans, nitric oxide can produce an innate immune reaction; lipid peroxidation by RNOS also causes bacteria cell death (Munir et al 2020; Pelgrift and Friedman, 2013).

Thus, Nitric oxide-releasing drugs – nitric oxide nanoparticles – with high Nitric Oxide dosage would slow down the protective enzymatic activities of the following: lactate dehydrogenase in MRSA and MSSA - Staphylococcus aureus; flavohemoglobin in staphylococcus aureus, escherichia coli, klebsiella pneumoniae, pseudomonas aeruginosa and salmonella typhimurium.

These bacteria have the natural ability to protect themselves from antibiotic effects but not in the presence of high nitric oxide delivered via nanoparticles. By hindering their growth, nitric oxide nanoparticles have a success rate with antibacterial actions especially those bacteria that are drug resistant. A dosage of 1.25-5mM of nitric oxide nanoparticles have been shown to destroy MRSA, escherichia coli, klebsiella pneumoniae, pseudomonas aeruginosa in culture (Munir et al 2020; Pelgrift and Friedman, 2013). Also, nitric oxide nanoparticles combat other infections such as candida albicans infections (Munir et al 2020; Pelgrift and Friedman, 2013).

- *Chitosan-based Nanoparticles (CHT-NPs):* These also use numerous mechanisms of action to combat antimicrobial resistance reducing the chances of resistance. The mechanisms are 1. The acetyl group removal from chitosan makes it positively charged which then produces an antimicrobial outcome when it interacts with negatively charged bacteria cells. This process increases cell membrane permeability. 2. Chitosan latches onto the bacteria DNA which prevents mRNA and protein transcription. 3. The activities of metalloproteins are reduced when Chitosan forms a heterocyclic bond with the metals. 4.Chitosan increases the healing process by promoting the release of fibroblast thus decreasing the likelihood of infection (Munir et al 2020).

Also, Chitosan-based nanoparticles have a higher success rate with gram negative bacteria because they are negatively charged and react with the positive charge of chitosan which increases cell permeability. Thus, antibiotic drugs can penetrate the cell wall membrane and provide effective treatment (Munir et al 2020).

- *Metal-based Nanoparticles:* Metal nanoparticles have various types of metal; these metals individually use more than one mechanism to destroy microbial development thus decreasing the potential for resistance

(Munir et al 2020; Pelgrift and Friedman, 2013). Some of the metal-based nanoparticles and how they prevent antimicrobial resistance are described below:

I. *Silver-based Nanoparticles (Ag NPs)* -: The positively charged ion of silver binds to the negatively charged cell wall and plasma membrane of the bacteria that contains sulfur and phosphorus. This process makes the cell wall of the bacteria porous and the cytoplasmic fluid flows out of the membrane leading to cell death. Gram negative bacteria may be affected more than gram positive because the former is negatively charged with a thinner cell wall and reacts with the positive charge of silver. A silver-based nanoparticle is beneficial in erythromycin-resistant Streptococcus pyogenes, ampicillin resistant escherichia coli and pseudomonas aeruginosa a multidrug-resistant bacterium ( Munir et al 2020; Pelgrift and Friedman, 2013).

II. *Zinc oxide-based nanoparticles (ZnO NPs):* These also use numerous mechanisms to combat drug resistance in bacteria. The mechanisms are the destruction of lipids and proteins contained in the cell membrane when zinc oxide nanoparticles bind to the membrane. This leads to increased permeability, cytoplasmic evacuation and cell death. Also, Zinc oxide nanoparticles form Zinc ions which react with oxygen causing cell mortality. Zinc oxide nanoparticles work to counter resistance of drug in methicillin resistant staphylococcus aureus (MRSA) (Pelgrift and Friedman, 2013).

### III. Copper-based nanoparticles (CuO NPs):

The mechanism of action is also multiple: copper forms a reactive compound with the amine and carboxyl group found in the bacteria. Also, at an elevated dose, it produces reactive oxygen species which prevents amino acid and DNA production. The higher the dosage of the copper-based nanoparticles the better the antibacterial effects. It has effects on bacteria such as escherichia coli and listeria monocytogenes (Munir et al 2020; Pelgrift and Friedman, 2013).

### IV. Magnesium-based nanoparticles (MgO

*NPs):* The mechanisms used to combat bacterial activity are: 1. The composition of a metal halide normally inhibits the activity of some enzymes within a bacterium. 2. Magnesium halogen produces lipid peroxidation in the membrane affecting the cytoplasmic activity, this occurs because of reactive oxygen species (ROS) activity. 3. It produces lipid peroxidation, reduction in PH and increase in membrane activity (Pelgrift and Friedman, 2013). Also, prevents the production of biofilms in escherichia coli and staphylococcus aureus (Munir et al 2020). Also, produces lipid peroxidation, reduction in PH and increase in membrane activity. 4. MgO absorbs halogen molecules to the surface which increases the antimicrobial activity – this action is unique to magnesium-based nanoparticles (Pelgrift and Friedman, 2013).

## 2.  Multiple antibiotics contained within a nanoparticle

Another way by which nanotechnology combats antimicrobial resistance is to put several antibiotics into a package of the nanoparticle. This method decreases the possibility of microbial resistance. Normally, the bacteria would require time for gene alteration necessary to fight the drugs but this method does not allow that. Packing different antibiotics into a nanoparticle promotes antimicrobial activity and treatment effectiveness. The success of this method supersedes that of using a single drug. An example of this application is seen when vancomycin is packed inside a chitosan nanoparticle and used to combat vancomycin resistant staphylococcus aureus (Munir et al 2020; Pelgrift and Friedman, 2013).

Moreover, to combat escherichia coli and vancomycin-resistant enterococcus (VRE) gold-based nanoparticles (Au NPs) is layered with ciprofloxacin antibiotic which improves antibacterial action and treatment outcome. This method also works to hinder and/or destroy MRSA, pseudomonas aeruginosa and proteus mirabilis bacteria. The use of combination treatment is more effective than the singular use of any of the treatments (Pelgrift and Friedman, 2013).

## 3. Using Nanoparticles to Combat Decreased Uptake and Increased Efflux

Liposomes and dendrimers are two nanoparticles that can be used to hinder the mechanism of action used by bacteria to inhibit drug efficacy – decreased drug uptake and increased efflux.

Structurally, the liposome is composed of a bi-lipid layer that is made up of components that help make membranes tough. Liposome evades the mechanism of decreased drug uptake because the bi-lipid layer helps the liposome bind rapidly to the plasma membrane and simultaneously release an elevated dosage of drug directly to the cytoplasm. Increased efflux mechanism is also avoided when an elevated amount of drug is delivered because it delivers an abundance of drug which overrides the effect of the pump action. Liposomes in combination with antibiotics produce quicker treatment results (Pelgrift and Friedman, 2013).

Dendrimers have large surface areas that help with antimicrobial activity. A positively charged surface area reacts with the negative charge of the bacterial membrane and increases permeability. Thus, dendrimers can access the bacterial cell, causing an overflow of the cytoplasm and cell mortality. This action overrides the decreased drug uptake mechanism adopted by antimicrobial resistant bacteria (Pelgrift and Friedman, 2013).

# 4. Prevention of Biofilm Formation Using Nanoparticles

Bacterial drug resistance can be inhibited when nanoparticles are used to prevent biofilm formation. Staphylococcus aurcus, escherichia coli, pseudomonas aeruginosa, candida albicans and staphylococcus epidermidis bacteria with biofilm formation can be destroyed using nanoparticles such as silver-based nanoparticle. It prevents the formation of biofilm and its destruction if already produced for example Staphylococcus aureus on a catheter is destroyed by silver-based nanoparticles increasing antimicrobial activity. Other nanoparticles that prevent or destroy biofilm are zinc oxide nanoparticles, gold-based nanoparticles and iron-based nanoparticles (Munir et al 2020).

## 5. Using Nanoparticles to Combat Intracellular Bacteria

Liposome, a nanoparticle, is minute in size, therefore, can penetrate the cellular space of bacteria to administer the antimicrobial drug directly within the cell destroying the bacteria. At an elevated dosage, it can destroy the bacteria before resistance formation. This method effectively combats mycobacterium tuberculosis (Pelgrift and Friedman, 2013).

## 6. Using Nanoparticles at the Site of Infection

Nanoparticles can be used at the site of infection either directly or indirectly. Direct target uses antibodies that latch onto antigens at the infection sites while indirect target uses tissue permeability caused by an outbreak of the inflammatory process at the site of infection. This method will cause minimal side effects while administering a high drug dosage. The site of infection will receive the antimicrobial drug combating the bacteria resistance. The administration of the drug at the site of infection can be controlled by a radio-frequency or image guided approach (Pelgrift and Friedman, 2013).

## Conclusion

Advancement in the use of nanotechnology to combat antimicrobial resistance will help alleviate the global health burden. Nanoparticles can destroy multiple drug-resistant bacteria because these bacteria have a single mechanism of action but Nanoparticles have multiple mechanisms of action and often work in combination with other treatment methods making it the first line of choice for antimicrobial drug resistance therapy. Nanotechnology allows for fast, safe and cost-saving treatment options for bacterial infections resistant to drugs and therapy.

# Chapter 7: The Promise of Phage Therapy

By: Dr. Austin Mardon & Amy Li

## What are Phages?

Bacteriophages (or phages for short) are viruses that infect bacteria. Phages' small size makes them easy to isolate and sequence genomically (Hatfull, 2008). Given the immensity of viral populations in the oceans, it is estimated that the total phage population is $10^{31}$ particles (Hatfull, 2008); it is also estimated that phages cause $10^{23}$ infections globally (Hatfull, 2008).

Phage genome size can be sorted into three groups. According to Hatfull (2008), a genome size of 30-50 kilo base pairs (kbp) makes up about 50% of all phages; 20% is <10 kbp; a size of 100-200 kbp makes up 6%. Phage structure and assembly of genes alone take up at least 15 kbp of their genome.

Phages have a distinct morphology. Phage tails consist of double stranded DNA (dsDNA) genomes (Hatfull, 2008). Phages' genomes are also enclosed in a protein shell/capsid and are semi-autonomous (Hobbs & Abedon, 2016). Based on their structure and sequence, phages are also sorted into families (Ganeshan & Hosseinidoust, 2019). The capsid makeup, the gene's chemical entities, and mRNA production are the defining criteria (Ganeshan & Hosseinidoust, 2019).

## Phages are genomically diverse

The changes in morphology largely contribute to the diversity in genomic organization and sequence differences; however, this diversity may hinder genetic transformation (Hatfull, 2008). One phage morphotype is the Siphovirus: about 20 kbp long in genome, it consists of head genes that include terminase subunits, portal proteins, capsid subunits; and tail genes that consist of a major tail subunit, a tape measure protein, and minor tail proteins (Hatfull, 2008). The tape measure protein is related to the phage tail's length, making up the largest gene in the genome (Hatfull, 2008).

Despite genome sizes differing by two-fold, phage genes can be found in different locations. For example, the lysis genes in some phages can be found adjacent to or between terminase genes; integration genes can be found in the center of the genome or near the tail genes (Hatfull, 2008). The diversity in gene arrangement makes phages unique and tailored to specific bacterial strains for therapy.

## Lytic Phages preferred for Phage Therapy

It is important to draw the distinction between lytic, lysogenic, and chronic phages. In the lytic cycle, phages adhere to the bacteria cell's receptor through ligands (sugar or protein) (Azam

& Tanji, 2019). Once bound to the receptors, phages inject their genome by sending internal capsid proteins into the host cell wall to create a pore for transfer (Ganeshan & Hosseinidoust, 2019). Afterwards, phage DNA is replicated; the host is lysed and phage progeny are released into the exterior (Ganeshan & Hosseinidoust, 2019). In phage therapy, scientists are only interested in using lytic phages.

Unlike lytic phages, lysogenic/temperate phages are not ideal for phage therapy. Once temperate phages' genomes are integrated into bacteria (becoming prophage), bacteria use prophage genes to survive, preventing subsequent phage infections (Jariah & Hakim, 2019). Some of these prophage genes include bacterial virulence factors; an example of a virulence factor is the Shiga-toxin found in *E. coli*, which causes severe diarrhoea (Jariah & Hakim, 2019). Virulence factors also cause bacterial cells to adhere to epithelial cells or platelets, increasing bacteria's infectivity (Jariah & Hakim, 2019). Temperate phages also facilitate transduction of antibiotic resistant genes to bacterial hosts, a mechanism exclusive to them (Jariah & Hakim, 2019). Chronic phages involve no lysing or integration of their genome into bacteria; they solely use the host to make more phages (Ganeshan & Hosseinidoust, 2019).

Based on their location and capsid state, phages can also be sorted into three categories: intracellular and not encapsidated; intracellular and not yet packaged within mature virions; and encapsidated and extracellular, where they are no longer bound to the host (Hobbs & Abedon, 2016).

# History of Phage Politics

In the past, the exact capabilities of phage therapy were still unknown. After being associated with treatment for diarrheal diseases, people thought that phage therapy was either revolutionary or just a waste of time (Summers, 2012).

In the early 1900s, the identification of phages was quite a historical, personal battle between two microbiologists who would try and one up each other. Félix d'Herelle, a French-Canadian microbiologist, believed that phages were a bacterial virus (Summers, 2012). Conversely, Frederick Twort, a British microbiologist, believed that phages were a lytic enzyme (Summers, 2012). Back then, most of the scientific community agreed with Twort.

The discovery of the electron microscope (EM) in the late 1930s quickly removed doubt from d'Herelle's claims (Summers, 2012). However, given that it was World War II, the bacteriophage EM images were not sent to America, and so France (including d'Herelle) received them first (Summers, 2012).

Another reason why the attitudes towards bacteriophages were controversial is because the scientific method was quite limited at the time. Back then, there was no conception of double-blind studies and use of statistics (Summers, 2012). Instead, scientists relied on clinical observations, anecdotal evidence, and controls from past experiments (Summers, 2012). Luckily, the development of literature reviews by the American Medical Association in the 30s and 40s helped with the ambiguity of bacteriophages (Summers, 2012). While three reports were published then, the studies had a weakness; the preparation of the phages as a polyvalent mixture chemically inactivated the phage, thus scientists were bound to get contradictory results (Summers, 2012).

Despite phage therapy discovery, American medicine in the 1940s found it much more convenient to use antibiotics and sulfa drugs (Summers, 2012). Unlike phages, antibiotics only required refrigeration for long shelf stability (Summers, 2012).

The political tensions between countries also did not help. During the post WWII period, Soviet knowledge was rejected by America. Since d'Herelle was employed in the Soviet Union, America would also reject d'Herelle's findings (Summers, 2012). Economic factors also marginalized phage therapy; unlike phage therapy, antibiotics were easier to prepare, more stable, were actually effective, and made huge profits (Summers, 2012).

In 1963, Gunther Stent, a part of a network of biologists, believed that phage therapy was impotent (Summers, 2012). Some of his reasons were: gastric juices in the mouth can digest the phage, making it ineffective, and the nature in which bacteria gain resistance is not favourable for phages (Summers, 2012). Believe it or not, Stent's arguments were more personal than scientific (Summers, 2012). Regardless of his lack of scientific evidence, he convinced people that phage therapy was irrelevant (Summers, 2012).

# How does Phage Therapy work?

Phage therapy targets a bacterial cell host, which can range between a bacterium within a single bacterial species to multiple bacterial genera (Chan et al., 2013). Phages also need to meet a bacterial target at a specific density to achieve the minimum inhibitory concentration; this is done in two ways: applying the phage directly at the site of infection, or systematically into the patient, such as by intravenous or subcutaneous administration (Chan et al., 2013).

## Phage cocktails

Rather than injecting single phages into the patient, scientists combine the most potent phages to create a phage 'cocktail' (Chan et al., 2013). In Gu et al.'s study, a phage cocktail was inserted into phage resistant bacteria; this study resulted in 100% recovery of bacteria in vivo, and 88% in vitro (as cited in Chan et al., 2013). In another study, Fillippov et al. introduced a mutation into phages to enhance their infectivity; as a result, Fillipov et al. found six receptors on eight of the phages studied and combined those phages to produce a cocktail (as cited in Chan et al., 2013). Fillippov et al.'s results showed that phage resistance was weakened in infected mice, increasing mice survival (as cited in Chan et al., 2013)

While phage cocktails are a great innovation for clinical medicine, combining too many phages in a cocktail might accidentally impact non-target bacteria instead (Chan et al., 2013). In addition, phage therapy itself may be too specific, since phages mainly target strains within a **single** bacterial species (Chan et al., 2013). One solution is to reduce the **complexity** of cocktails, since the host range is still limited and phage susceptibility of pathogenic bacteria may change overtime (Chan et al., 2013).

## Approaches to designing phage cocktails

There are two approaches to formulating phage therapy. One way is to assemble the phage at the time of drug authentication (prêt-à-porter) or allow changes to the drug development process (sur-mesure) (Chan et al., 2013).

The prêt-à-porter method may be disadvantageous, since it implies that one single cocktail is designed to have an effect on multiple pathogens that cause a particular infection; this is often termed as the Western model of drug development (Chan et al., 2013). This type of method would be suitable if consistency is constantly met in drug formulation (Chan et al., 2013).

A middle ground between both approaches would be to make multiple cocktails that each contain several single phages that target one bacterial species (Chan et al., 2013). In this way, if cocktails are used against an infection and are ineffective, the cocktail can then be followed up against other bacterial species (Chan et al., 2013).

When choosing phages, it would be desirable to choose from a 'cocktail bank'. This bank would use fewer phage types, however the development of this bank comes at a huge cost (Chan et al., 2013). Another middle ground would be to use a single cocktail that can be modified later on; for instance, phages that target the most pathogenic strains can be added (Chan et al.,

2013).

Considering the elements of personalized medicine, phage therapy could tailor their cocktails to individual patients' needs (Chan et al., 2013). However, given the gaps in knowledge of bacteria-phage interactions, meeting this goal could be lengthy. In addition, the 'personalized' approach can only provide information on which phages are suitable, without any **proof** of their activity (Chan et al., 2013).

## Phages interact with Human Immune System

Phages are found virtually everywhere in the human body, namely the human intestine (Jariah & Hakim, 2019). To locate to other regions of the body, phages require receptor binding to membranes, which leads to signal transduction and endocytosis in cells (Jariah & Hakim, 2019). In particular, the phage-related killing of bacteria triggers the innate immune response; the aftermath is the production of endotoxins and lipopolysaccharide (LPS), which should be avoided in future preparations of phage (Jariah & Hakim, 2019).

A pharmacological issue of phage therapy is how to avoid harming the host immune system. This can be achieved by isolating the phage properly, modification to the phage, and alternate routes of phage delivery, such as oral administration (Chan et al., 2013).

Together, the immune system and phages eliminate bacterial pathogens. Phages accomplish this by: triggering bacterial phagocytosis by macrophages, coating the bacterial cell to increase the availability of bacteria to phagocytes, and the co-presence of phagocytosis and the lytic cycle (Jariah & Hakim, 2019). One drawback is that there are reduced levels of reactive oxygen species (ROS) observed in phages (Jariah & Hakim, 2019); ROS is produced to help eliminate bacterial pathogens.

Toll-like receptors are pathogen-associated molecules that the innate immune system recognizes. However, the link between phages and toll-like receptors is limited and requires further study (Jariah & Hakim, 2019). On the other hand, there is an interaction between phage receptors and the production of cytokines (molecules secreted by cells of the immune system); phages induce anti-inflammatory effects by hindering nuclear transcription factors found in the immune system, as well as tumour necrosis factor α (TNF-α) and interleukin 6 (IL-6) (Jariah & Hakim, 2019). Notwithstanding, the precise mechanism of phages inducing anti-inflammatory properties remains to be solved (Jariah & Hakim, 2019).

Phages are also involved in humoral/B-cell immunity. In particular, IgG and IgM antibodies were found bound to phage tails (Jariah & Hakim, 2019). To neutralize phages, it requires the complement system (part of an immune system that helps clear pathogens), leading to higher secretion of anti-phage antibodies, and overall lower phage activity (Jariah & Hakim, 2019). Understanding the neutralization of phages, it is important to choose phages that will not trigger a huge immune response, otherwise the phages' effectiveness and activity will decrease (Jariah & Hakim, 2019).

The way phage therapy is administered also impacts B-cell

immunity. In one case, oral administration resulted in a lower production of IgA and IgG antibodies (Jariah & Hakim, 2019). Certain phage proteins also trigger humoral immunity moreso than others. For example, Hoc and gp12 proteins particularly elevate production of IgG and IgA antibodies in the blood and the gut than other phage proteins (Jariah & Hakim, 2019).

# PHAGE THERAPY'S CURRENT PROGRESS

## Clinical Studies on Phage Therapy

Several studies examined a reduction of pathogenic bacteria by a factor of $10^5$, while other studies saw a reduction by a single ten-fold (Chan et al., 2013). One study by Wright et al. was the first double-blind Phase I/II clinical trial, but it had weaknesses: the observations relied on a visual analog scale; the physician used subjective findings; and ear swabs were obtained to get semi-quantitative results (Chan et al., 2013). Nonetheless, the phage treatment group had an overall 50% reduction in the pathogen; the placebo had a 20% reduction (Chan et al., 2013).

While the preparation of phages were consistent, for future studies it is imperative that phages be propagated separately, purified, and mixed prior to treatment (Chan et al., 2013). In several cocktails, viral interference was observed: interference prevents secondary infection of a subsequent phage. From these studies, scientists learnt to: elucidate phage formulations and their benefits, and prevent phage-resistant mutants during treatment (Chan et al., 2013).

## Is Phage Therapy acceptable in Western Medicine?

The single-cocktail modifiable approach has the advantage of not requiring to start over the whole process of drug approval (Chan et al., 2013). In addition, phage therapy is not inherently dangerous to humans, and less in need of inactivation. Nonetheless, they still require characterization prior to use in therapy (Chan et al., 2013); this may be an inconvenience for Western medicine. Luckily, the field of bioinformatics should determine phage properties and which phages to avoid (Chan et al., 2013).

To improve the tedious process of phage characterization, phage isolate approval should be based on predefined, specific criteria rather than a lengthy approval process that involves clinical considerations and trials (Chan et al., 2013). The criteria should include: how the bacterium is treated, the chemical entities of the phage formulations (pH, preservatives, etc.) (Chan et al., 2013).

If not acceptable in Western medicine, phage therapy may play a role in replacing biopesticides. Similar to phages, biopesticides are less toxic than their counterparts, carrying fewer risks, and less time to register for formal use (Chan et al., 2013). Therefore, perhaps phages can be used in agriculture as antibacterial biopesticides (Chan et al., 2013).

The current obstacle is how to integrate phage therapy into existing regulatory rules and into economic models that control distribution and usage of antibacterial molecules (Chan et al., 2013). As of right now, phage therapy seems to succeed in regions that are regulatorily friendly, and where the profits are very small (Chan et al., 2013). Furthermore, we need more published studies on phage therapy to inform the scientific field, as well as a stronger need for prêt-à-porter phage cocktails (Chan et al., 2013).

## Bacterial Evolution's Impact on Phage Therapy Development

Depending on the rate of bacterial evolution, the occurrence of phage-resistant bacteria may be inevitable; this is not necessarily a bad thing (Jariah & Hakim, 2019). When gaining phage-resistance, bacteria also lose important genes crucial for their fitness and consequently, losing their bacterial virulence (Jariah & Hakim, 2019). This setback also gives time for the human immune system to harness a response towards bacteria, reinforcing the synergy between the immune system and phages (Jariah & Hakim, 2019).

As of right now, prevention of phage resistance is the best measure to take. Scientists can achieve this by: creating large populations of phages in the initial stages, achieving short pre-infectious periods, and obtaining more general host ranges (Jariah & Hakim, 2019). Phages within a cocktail should also target various components of the bacterial cell surface to prevent phage competition; cocktails tailored to the patient should be used to prevent the number of phages used (Jariah & Hakim, 2019).

# Phage Therapy vs. Antibiotics: The Pros and Cons

There is much heated discussion about phage therapy as an alternative to antibiotics. The advantages and disadvantages of phage therapy are outlined below, with the information derived from Loc-Carrillo & Abedon (2011).

## Main Advantages of Phage Therapy

- The lethality of phage therapy is more enhanced than antibiotics
- Auto "dosing"
  - Phages can increase their number where hosts are found
- Low toxicity
  - Phages are composed of nucleic acids and protein, making them less toxic
- They do not affect the normal flora, owing to their high host specificity
- Lower incidence of bacterial resistance, once again because of their host specificity
- Antibiotic resistance does not share similarities with phage resistance
  - Therefore, phages can be used to treat bacterial infections that resist antibiotics
- Phages are easy to isolate from target bacteria and are non-toxic
- Phages have a wide range of formulations and

application types

- ○ Can form cocktails to result in a broader spectrum of activity
- ○ Application types include: creams, liquids, solids, etc.
- Phages can destroy biofilms more effectively, due to lysing bacterial layers one at a time


## Other advantages of Phage Therapy

- A single dose may only be required, considering the auto dosing effect
  - ○ Convenient, but to be safe, a single dose is not advised
- Phages transferring between subjects may hold agricultural uses
- A lower phage dose could improve cost efficacy
  - ○ Improves product safety because phages only increase in concentration **if bacteria is actively being killed**
- Discarding phages will only impact a small portion of environmental bacteria
  - ○ Once exposed to sunlight or exterior temperatures, phages not used to those conditions will be easily decayed
- Phages carry no misuses thus far
  - ○ Antibiotics on the other hand are often misused. Examples include: empirical use

without knowing the consequences on serious infections, use in animal feeds
- Phages have no ethical issues since they are natural products
- Phages are economically worthwhile and cheap to produce
  - ◦ Phage purification is cheap as well

## Disadvantages of Phage Therapy

- While non-temperate phages are preferred, temperate phages still pose a risk
  - ◦ Temperate phages cannot avoid bacterial defenses and fail to replicate properly
- Phage characterization can be costly
  - ◦ Characterization involves their morphology, protein identification, genotypes, full-genome sequencing
- The narrow host range limits phage treatment especially during preliminary treatment (prior to identifying the pathogen)
- While phages are not entirely unique, it is not a reason to reject page therapy
  - ◦ Nonetheless, phage therapy behaves much differently than antibiotics
    - ▪ Right now, the medical field is still unfamiliar with phages
- A weakness in the field would be the lack of phase III clinical trials, and double-blinded

studies for phage therapy
- ◦ And consequently, a lack of funding

# Phages can adapt to Bacterial Defense Mechanisms

Bacteria use a variety of mechanisms to evade phage infection. Bacteria can either evade infection at the stage of phage DNA absorption or after absorption (Azam & Tanji, 2019).

During absorption, bacteria can alter phage receptors so that phages no longer bind; phages can **counter** this by acquiring point mutations in their receptor binding proteins, thus latching onto a new receptor rather than the older one. In addition, phages can create degrading enzymes that target the protective wall of phage-resistant bacteria (Azam & Tanji, 2019). Phages can also evade the bacteria's phase variation: phase variation is the bacteria adapting to their environment, requiring no mutations (Azam & Tanji, 2019). Phages do this by modifying receptor binding proteins that can interact with the host's surface at any point in time (Azam & Tanji, 2019).

After injection of phage DNA into the host cell, bacteria can cleave the DNA through their innate or adaptive systems (Azam & Tanji, 2019). In particular, bacteria have two enzymes that facilitate anti-phage defense, termed the **restriction-modification (R-M) system**: restriction endonucleases and methyl transferases (Azam & Tanji, 2019). The former cuts phage DNA while the latter methylates bacterial DNA for protection from the endonuclease (Azam & Tanji, 2019). Phages can avoid the restriction of endonuclease by not having the endonuclease site in their genome, or having their DNA methylated to escape endonuclease cleavage (Azam & Tanji, 2019).

Bacteria also use a CRISPR-Cas system to evade phage infection. Essentially, bacteria incorporate fragments of foreign DNA into their genome or the CRISPR loci (Azam & Tanji, 2019). The DNA sequences inserted into the CRISPR array act as a recognition site to prevent invading phages that carry the same DNA segment (Jariah & Hakim, 2019). Once CRISPR-RNAs are synthesized, they act as a guide and create a complex with a Cas protein to cleave phage DNA (Jariah & Hakim, 2019). Phages avoid this system by obtaining point mutations in the PAM region (a sequence found in the phage that Cas9 targets) that recognizes Cas9, inhibiting the system (Azam & Tanji, 2019).

Bacteria have also adapted to produce their own mature phage virions, rather than ones originating from invading phage virions (Azam & Tanji, 2019). This mechanism is encoded in a region called the phage inducible chromosomal island: this island allows for the production of smaller capsids, preventing phage packaging and phage gene inactivation (Azam & Tanji, 2019). As a result, the phage dies and releases virions that contain DNA from the islands, into adjacent cells, rather than their own DNA (Azam & Tanji, 2019). However, it is speculated that phages use the CRISPR-Cas system in their own genome to avoid this defense mechanism (Azam & Tanji, 2019).

Abortive infection is an extreme method for eliminating phages (Figure 5). This mechanism kills the bacterial host cell, preventing infection of specific strains of phage (Azam & Tanji, 2019). Phages counter this attack by producing antitoxins against bacterial toxins (Azam & Tanji, 2019).

## Conclusion

Despite the controversial opinions of phage therapy in the past, the advantages of phage therapy highlight its potential to replace antibiotics. The main pros of phage therapy are: its low toxicity, high host specificity, and auto "dosing" effect. Regardless, the arms race between phages and bacteria will persist for generations.

It would be beneficial to focus on the prevention of phage-resistant bacteria, and improve methods of phage characterization and phage cocktail design. Given the advances in technology and bioinformatics, these issues may be resolved soon. As well, more publications and clinical studies on phage therapy will spread awareness and help increase funding for this promising field in microbiology.

# Chapter 8: Bacteriocins for Multidrug Resistance Therapy

By: Dr. Austin Mardon & Sriraam Sivachandran

## Antibiotics & Antibiotics Resistance

Through medicinal developmental history, various treatment options have attempted to treat bacterial infections. The development of antibiotics was seen as a success as they were becoming more viable options to treat various bacterial infections. One of the most famous antibiotics is penicillin, which was first released in 1941 (CDC, 2020). An antibiotic that was released recently was ceftazidime-avibactam, which was released in 2015 (CDC, 2020). The actual success of antibiotics can be seen in statistics such as life span. In the United States, the life span increased from 56.4 years old to 80 years old due to the emergence of antibiotics (Ventola, 2015). However, there has been an increased number of people suffering from diseases due to antibiotic resistant bacterial infections. Antibiotic resistance occurs when bacteria and fungi gain resistance against specific drugs that would usually eliminate them (CDC, 2020). There has been a significant increase in the number of antibiotic resistant bacteria and fungi. Every year, at least 2.8 million people are infected and more than 35,000 people die in the United States because of antibiotic-resistant bacteria or fungi (CDC, 2020).

## Antibiotic Resistance Mechanism

It is important to understand the various mechanisms in which bacteria and fungi may attempt to resist the effects of antibiotics. It is also important to understand the causes of the increasing number of antibiotic resistant bacteria and fungi. These bacteria or fungi have the ability to use specific resistance mechanisms against drugs. The Centers for Disease Control and Prevention outlines five common resistance mechanisms. Firstly, some bacteria and fungi can restrict access of the antibiotic by changing or lowering the number of entryways (CDC, 2020). Secondly, some bacteria and fungi have the ability to get rid of the antibiotic drugs that have already entered the cell by using pumps in their cell wall (CDC, 2020). Another mechanism used involves the usage of enzymes and other proteins that can destroy the antibiotic (CDC, 2020). Some bacteria and fungi can develop new cell processes that will allow them to bypass the drugs' effects (CDC, 2020). Lastly, some bacteria and fungi can change the antibiotic's target so the drug cannot recognize it as the true target (CDC, 2020).

The ability for bacteria or fungi to resist antibiotic drugs does not appear all of a sudden. There are certain reasons as to why certain bacteria and fungi become antibiotic-resistant. One of the most well-known causes of the development of antibiotic resistance is the overuse of the antibiotic drugs. There is a direct correlation between antibiotic consumption and certain resistant bacteria strains (Ventola, 2015). Horizontal gene transfer is the process in which antibiotic resistance is transferred between different bacterial species (Ventola, 2015). When looking specifically at the United States, some states have more prescribed antibiotics than the total population, which suggests that each person has more than one antibiotic prescription (Ventola, 2015). Unfortunately, in certain countries, the availability of antibiotics is heightened because of the lack of regulations and the online availability (Ventola, 2015).

Another cause of increased antibiotic resistant bacteria and fungi is the inappropriate prescribing of antibiotics. In 30% to 50% of cases, the treatment indication, choice of antibiotic, or duration of antibiotic therapy is done incorrectly (Ventola, 2015). A study done by Bartlett et al showed that out of 17,435 patients that were hospitalized with pneumonia, a pathogen was identified in only 7.6% of the patients (Bartlett et al., 2013). Furthermore, up to 60% of the antibiotics that are prescribed in intensive care units have been deemed unnecessary. When looking more into the mechanism of inappropriate prescribing, it has the ability to subject patients to complications of antibiotic therapy. Improper antibiotic concentrations can actually commence the start of antibiotic resistance due to specific mechanisms that can affect gene changes. Some examples of these mechanisms are gene expression, horizontal gene transfer, and mutagenesis. When gene expression changes occur, there is an increased chance of virulence. If there is increased mutagenesis and horizontal gene transfer, there is increased promotion of antibiotic resistance and spread (Ventola, 2015).

Increased agricultural use of antibiotics is another cause of increased antibiotic resistant bacteria and fungi. Various food companies utilise antibiotics in animals in order to promote growth and prevent infection (Ventola, 2015). When these animals are treated with these antibiotics, the overall health of the animals is supposed to improve and give better quality meat (Ventola, 2015). Specifically, in the United States about 80% of antibiotics that are usually sold are used in animals (Ventola, 2015). Unfortunately, when humans consume meat products that have been treated with antibiotics, antibiotic resistance genes can transfer to humans. This process actually occurs in three steps. Firstly, the antibiotics in the meat that humans consume may have the ability to suppress certain bacteria and that allows antibiotic resistant bacteria to thrive in that environment (Ventola, 2015). Next, the antibiotic resistant bacteria is transferred to humans that actually eat the antibiotic treated meat (Ventola, 2015). Lastly, if humans ingest these resistant bacteria, there may be unfavourable consequences to their health. Antibiotics are not only used in animals as the practice of antibiotics in plants is well known. For example, even though animals are given antibiotics, up to 90% are released through urine and feces which goes into the soil and consequently various runoffs (Ventola, 2015); another example would be when farmers spray certain antibiotics in fruit trees (Ventola, 2015).

Another cause for the increased number of antibiotic resistant bacteria and fungi is the lack of new antibiotics. Even though scientists continue to attempt to develop new antibiotics, there is an evident lack of results.  From 1980 to 1999, there were 52 new antibiotics that were developed and approved.  However, from 2000 to 2014, there were only 13 new antibiotics approved (Ventola, 2015).  An argument could be made that there were more antibiotics approved in the past because there was more potential for discovery of new antibiotics.  However, it can also be said that there are more tools available to scientists today that should help with the development of new antibiotics.

## Bacteriocins

Bacteriocins are antimicrobial peptides that are produced by bacteria (Yang et al., 2014).  These bacteriocins have large diversity because they are very abundant (Yang et al., 2014).  One of the main and most promising abilities of bacteriocins is its ability to kill harmful bacteria.  This advanced ability allows bacteriocins to maintain population and limit the number of competitors, which leads to an increased chance of nutrient uptake and better habitability in a specific environment.  It is important to note that bacteriocins are actually ribosomally synthesized, and are harmless to the human body and its environment for the most part (Yang et al., 2014).

## Classification of Bacteriocins

Bacteriocins can be classified based on the bacteria that is actually producing them.  The two types of bacteria that produce bacteriocins are gram-negative bacteria and gram-positive bacteria and within this classification, there are different bacteriocins with different properties and mechanisms.

1. Gram-negative bacteria can cause various diseases in the human body to different organ systems (Oliveira & Reygaert, 2021).

   - One type of bacteriocins from gram-negative bacteria is colicin. Colicins are produced by bacteria and are antibacterial proteins which have the ability to kill bacterial strains to limit the number of environmental competitors. Colicins are produced by *E. coli* and have been used for a long time to understand bacteriocins and their evolution. Colicins mainly have two important functions: they have the ability to form pores in the bacterial wall and they are able to degrade nucleic acid structures (Simons et al., 2020). The formation of pores in the bacterial wall can lead to cytoplasmic compounds leaking, and it destabilises the electrochemical gradient due to ion loss. This can only be done by certain colicins (A, B, K, N, E1, Ia, Ib). This ultimately leads to cell death. On the other hand, some colicins can destroy the DNA and RNA of the harmful bacteria (E2 – E9) which eliminates all the nucleic material of the harmful bacteria (Yang et al., 2014). Colicins have three different domains: amino-terminal translocation (T) domain, central receptor-binding (R) domain, and the carboxy-terminal cytotoxic (C) domain. The T domain is involved in the process of transfer across the outer membrane of a cell using the translocator protein.

The R domain is actually located with the bacterial outer membrane receptor and the C domain has antibacterial activity. If a specific bacterium has the colicin recognition receptor on its outer membrane surface, the colicins are able to enter the cell. Once the colicin is transported into the bacterium, it will kill the bacteria. The different types of colicins use different protein systems to enter the outer membrane of the harmful bacteria (Yang et al., 2014).

- The second group of bacteriocins that come from gram-negative bacteria is microcins. Microcins have a lower molecular weight compared to colicins. Precursor peptides, N-terminal leader peptides and core peptides all produce microcins. Similar to colicins, microcins have different mechanisms that can be used to fight and kill harmful bacteria. For example, microcins can create pores in the bacterial wall, and they also have similar functionality to DNase and RNase. Furthermore, microcins are able to inhibit DNA replication and protein synthesis (Yang et al., 2014). Within the microcins, there are two subclasses: Subclass I and Subclass II. Subclass I microcins are categorized as post-translationally modified bacteriocins. These microcins have a lower molecular weight than Subclass II microcins which are known as minimally modified peptides (Simons et al., 2020).

2. The other type of bacteria that produces bacteriocins are gram-positive bacteria. Bacteria are deemed to be gram-positive because they turn a specific colour when they undergo a staining method (Sizar & Unakal, 2021).

- There are three classes of gram-positive bacteriocins. Class I is also known as lantibiotics and post-translationally modified bacteriocins. Bacteriocins in this group form numerous ring structures and are stable underheat, pH, and proteolysis because they feature many diverse amino acids. A modification such as the addition of certain amino acids is done post-translationally due to processes such as dehydration and cyclization. This group is further divided into two subclasses. Subclass Ia consist of positively charged elongated peptides that are involved in the formation of the pores in the bacterial wall. On the other hand, subclass Ib lantibiotics are negatively charged, and their shape is globular and stiff. These bacteriocins have the ability to inhibit enzymes that are used by the harmful bacteria (Simons et al., 2020).

- The second class of bacteriocins from gram-positive bacteria is known as non-lantibiotics or class II. These bacteriocins are opposite to lantibiotics as they do not have any unusual amino acids. However, similar to lantibiotics, they are small, and they also have heat stability. These bacteriocins have the ability to destabilize or permeabilize responses toward the bacterial wall, and share similar functionality with other bacteriocins because they can also cause the formation of pores in the bacterial wall. Non-antibiotics can be divided into four subclasses. The first subclass, subclass IIa, has a linear structure with disulfide bridges. Subclass IIb are deemed to be two-peptide bacteriocins which are classified as alpha and beta. Both of these peptides are needed in order for those specific bacteriocins to share antibiotic functionality. Subclass IIc are small bacteriocins that include one or two cysteine residues. Lastly, subclass IId has the ability to gather all the different non-lantibiotic bacteriocins (Simons et al., 2020).

- The third class of bacteriocins from gram-positive bacteria are simply called class III bacteriocins. These bacteriocins are larger in size compared to the previous two classes. Class III shows some enzymatic activity, along with antibacterial activity which ultimately disrupts the bacterial wall (Simons et al., 2020).

- The last class of bacteriocins from gram-positive bacteria are categorized as class IV bacteriocins. These bacteriocins have carbohydrates and lipids incorporated into their structure which helps with the disruption of the cell wall (Simons et al., 2020).

* * *

## Bacteriocins and Multidrug Resistance

Due to the increase of antibiotic resistant bacteria and fungi, there has been a search for different methods and processes that may facilitate the fight against more advanced bacteria. An example of one of those methods is indeed bacteriocins. One of the key advantages of using bacteriocins is the fact that they have slightly different functionality compared to certain antibiotics (Soltani et al., 2021). If bacteria are able to resist the antibiotics, it is very likely that cross-resistance does not occur because the antibiotics have different functions compared to the bacteriocins, and certain bacteriocins have a variety of different and effective functions to combat harmful bacteria. Another advantage to using bacteriocins against harmful bacteria is the fact that bacteriocins can be combined together or combined with other antibiotics. This results in a wider array of mechanisms that can be used to fight against harmful bacteria, and it reduces the chance of the bacteria developing resistance (Soltani et al., 2021). There are certain examples of different bacteriocins that can combat antibiotic resistant bacteria or fungi. These include but are not limited to nisin, bacteriocin PJ4, bacteriocin VJ13, and etc.

## Conclusion

The fight against antibiotic resistant bacteria and fungi is ongoing and a critical battle. Although there has been an increase in scientific advancement, certain bacteria have become resistant to some of the antibiotics that are developed, and it is important to find alternative methods to counteract this phenomenon. Even though the use of bacteriocins is a relatively novel approach, with more research and development, bacteriocins may be the next best way to combat antibiotic resistant bacteria and fungi without harming the human body.

# Chapter 9: Algae as a Novel Source of Antibiotic Discovery

By: Dr. Austin Mardon & Margaret Wa Yan Choi

## Introduction

The alarming phenomenon of increased antibiotic resistance needs to be properly addressed. To overcome antibiotic resistance, novel antibacterial or antimicrobial agents need to be developed. It is the goal of scientists and researchers to identify environmental friendly, sustainable, and bioactive compounds from natural products (Parsaeimehr and Lutzu, 2016). As the marine environment houses diverse ecosystems and microorganisms, many marine organisms have evolved to defend themselves from infections caused by bacteria that reside in ocean waters, it is therefore of no surprise that marine organisms would be explored for their antimicrobial potential (Shannon and Abu-Ghannam, 2016). Among these many organisms, algae is one notable example, which researchers have found to have the potential of being a reliable source of antimicrobial compounds (Pérez et al., 2016).

Algae are a polyphyletic, broad group of eukaryotic organisms that can be unicellular or multicellular (Parsaeimehr and Lutzu, 2016; Bhowmick et al., 2020). They can live in isolated forms as well as in organized colonies, and are often found in freshwater, marine water, sea shores, and rock surfaces (Bhowmick et al., 2020). Marine algae can be classified into three major groups based on their pigmentation and chemical composition, these three groups are: (1) Phaeophyceae (brown algae), (2) Rhodophyceae (red algae), and (3) Chlorophyceae (green algae) (Xu et al., 2017). Different algal species may also differ in their ways of obtaining energy or food (Parsaeimehr and Lutzu, 2016). Most species of algae are photosynthetic or autotrophic, meaning that they can produce their own food using light, water, carbon dioxide, or other chemicals (Parsaeimehr and Lutzu, 2016; Pérez et al., 2016; National Geographic, n.d.). Some other species such as *Cochlodinium polykrikoides*, are mixotrophic, and can gain energy from both photosynthesis and the uptake of organic carbon (Parsaeimehr and Lutzu, 2016). There are also species like *Crypthecodinium cohnii*, which have very limited or no photosynthetic activity (Parsaeimehr and Lutzu, 2016).

Algae, as mentioned above, inhabit harsh marine environments (Lefranc et al., 2019). Marine organisms including algae are constantly exposed to osmotic stress, high levels of ultraviolet (UV) light and salinity (Shannon and Abu-Ghannam, 2016). In addition, these organisms would have to face threats of infection by resident pathogenic bacteria (Hughes and Fenical, 2010). To cope with such conditions, algae produce complex compounds and metabolites that can present antiviral, antiprotozoal, antifungal, and antibacterial properties (Lefranc et al., 2019;

Pérez et al., 2016). Many of these substances isolated from different algal species have been identified to be polysaccharides, fatty acids, pigments, polyphenols, alkaloids, terpenes, and peptides etc (Bhowmick et al., 2020; Pérez et al., 2016). Previous studies have shown that these substances made by algae demonstrate greater antibacterial efficacy than those from terrestrial sources, and it is suggested that this is due to the greater number of bacterial cells in aquatic environments compared to in the air (Shannon and Abu-Ghannam, 2016). A variety of algal metabolites exhibit potential antimicrobial activity, and because algae can be cultured in high volumes, they are considered a very attractive source of compounds useful for novel antibiotic discovery amid the crisis of increased antibiotic resistance (Bhowmick et al., 2020; Pérez et al., 2016).

## Algae with Antimicrobial Properties

Different algae produce different algal metabolites with varying antimicrobial activities (Bhowmick et al., 2020). Some have antimicrobial activity against a wider array of bacteria, while some are against a narrower range of bacteria or microbes (Bhowmick et al., 2020). For instance, *Saccharina longicruris*, a marine algae, has demonstrated effective antibacterial activity only against *Staphylococcus aureus*, a gram-positive bacterium that can cause skin, urinary tract, and pulmonary infections (Bhowmick et al., 2020; Taylor and Unakal, 2020; Beaulieu et al., 2015). However, it is not effective against gram-negative bacteria (Bhowmick et al., 2020). In contrast, *Nizamuddinia zanardinii*, another marine algae, can target several types of gram-negative bacteria including *Escherichia coli* (*E. coli*) and

Pseudom*onas aeruginosa* (*P. aeruginosa*), but has no effect on any of the gram-positive bacteria (Bhowmick et al., 2020; Alboofetileh et al., 2019).

Nevertheless, there are plenty of other algae with antimicrobial activity against both gram-positive and gram-negative bacteria (Bhowmick et al., 2020). One remarkable example is *Chlorella vulgaris*, in fact, algal extracts' antibacterial potential was first reported in a study of *Chlorella vulgaris* (Bhowmick et al., 2020; Pratt et al., 1944). *Chlorella vulgaris* can produce a substance named chlorellin, which is capable of inhibiting the growth of both gram-positive and gram-negative bacteria including *Streptococcus pyogenes* (*S. pyogenes*), *Staphylococcus aureus* (*S. aureus*), *Bacillus subtilis* (*B. subtilis*), and *Pseudomona aeruginosa* (*P. aeruginosa*) (Bhowmick et al., 2020; Pratt et al., 1944). Another example is *Turbinaria triquetra*, which has been proven effective in inhibiting multiple gram-positive and gram-negative bacteria, one of which being Methicillin-resistant *Staphylococcus aureus* (MRSA), a strain of *S. aureus* that is resistant to commonly used antibiotics (Bhowmick et al., 2020; Al-Judaibi, 2014; Pantosti and Venditti, 2009). As seen in these examples, algae indeed bear great potential in antibiotics discovery.

## Polysaccharides from Algae

Polysaccharides are polymers containing long chains of monosaccharides connected through glycosidic bonds (Holesh et al., 2020). They serve as major structural components that make up cell walls of marine algae, providing rigidity and strength

(Bhowmick et al., 2020; Pérez et al., 2016). It should be noted that in these cell walls of marine algae, the polysaccharides are often sulphated, whereas cell walls in plants are not (Bhowmick et al., 2020). Algae contain an array of polysaccharides, including alginic acid, alginates, carrageenans, agar, laminarrans, fucoidans, ulvans, and their derivatives (Pérez et al., 2016). Recently, numerous polysaccharides have been isolated from marine algae for applications in the fields of functional foods, pharmaceuticals, and cosmetics (Xu et al., 2017). Some of these polysaccharides possess antimicrobial activity, which usually correlates with different factors such as their molecular weight, charge density, structures, types, and features of glycosidic linkages (Pérez et al., 2016; Xu et al., 2017). Moreover, a number of marine algal polysaccharides not only have antimicrobial activities, but also anticoagulant, antioxidant, antitumor, and immunomodulatory activities, making algae a very appealing source of medicine to explore (Xu et al., 2017).

Many algae contain sulphated polysaccharides with antibacterial activity. For example, polysaccharides isolated from *Gracilaria ornata*, a marine alga, have antibacterial activity against *E. coli*. Polysaccharides from another marine alga, *Chaetomorpha aerea, is* effective against gram-positive *B. subtilis* and *Micrococcus luteus* (*M. luteus*), as well as the drug-resistant *S. aureus* (Bhowmick et al., 2020). Laminarin, a polysaccharide extracted from the Irish brown marine alga *Laminaria hyperborea* and *Ascophyllum nodosum* have demonstrated significant inhibition of *S. aureus*, *E. coli*, *Listeria monocytogenes*, and *salmonella typhimurium* (Shannon and Abu-Ghannam, 2016; Bhowmick et al., 2020).

Algal polysaccharides with antimicrobial activities usually target the DNA of bacterial cells (Bhowmick et al., 2020). The mechanism of action is proposed to involve glycoprotein receptors in the polysaccharides, which can bind to the molecules on the bacterial cell wall, membrane, and nucleic acids (Bhowmick et al., 2020). The interactions between these receptors and the molecules located on the bacterial cells would then lead to disorganization of the membrane structure, loss of membrane permeability, leakage of proteins, and dysfunctionality of bacterial DNA, ultimately resulting in the bacterial cell death (Shannon and Abu-Ghannam, 2016; Bhowmick et al., 2020; He et al., 2010).

## Polyphenols from Algae

Polyphenols are one of most important compounds to consider when determining the biomedical importance of algae (Besednova et al., 2020). They are characterized by an aromatic ring with hydroxyl groups attached (Pérez et al., 2016; Bhowmick et al., 2020). They are highly hydrophilic secondary metabolites produced by algae and many other plants, but are not directly involved in primary processes like photosynthesis, cell division, or reproduction (Besednova et al., 2021, Pérez et al., 2016). Instead, polyphenols play roles in defense against ultraviolet radiation or invasion by pathogens (Pandey and Rizvi, 2009). Polyphenols are very abundant in algae, and as polyphenols have highly conjugated systems and hydroxyl groups, they contribute heavily to algae's relatively high antioxidant property (Pérez et al., 2016; Bhowmick et al., 2020; Tsao, 2010).

The antioxidant properties are not the only potential benefits these algal polyphenols offer. In fact, polyphenols derived from algae also display potential for antibacterial, antifungal, anti-inflammatory, antimalaria, and anticancer properties (Bhowmick et al., 2020). This variety of properties can be attributed to polyphenols' ability to interact with multiple sites on bacterial cells (Bhowmick et al., 2020). Polyphenols can bind to surface adhesive molecules, increase membrane permeability, fluidity, disrupt osmotic pressure, and inhibit enzymes of metabolic pathways, thereby killing bacterial cells (Bhowmick et al., 2020).

There are multiple types of polyphenols found in algae with antibacterial activity, it is also known that they generally target or disrupt metabolic pathways of bacterial cells (Bhowmick et al., 2020). One of them is phlorotannins (Bhowmick et al., 2020). Phlorotannins consist of polymeric units of phloroglucinol (1,3,5-trihydroxybenzene) and are produced in the acetate-malonate pathway (Bhowmick et al., 2020). They kill bacterial cells by binding to the membrane enzymes as well as those that are essential to metabolic pathways, and by directly inhibiting the oxidative phosphorylation, which cumulatively induce cell lysis in the end (Bhowmick et al., 2020; Wang et al., 2009). The hydroxyl groups also take part in such interactions as they enhance the ability of phlorotannins to bind with amide groups of bacterial proteins through hydrophobic interactions and hydrogen binding, further improving their efficacy in killing the bacterial cells. One example of phlorotannins exhibiting antibacterial properties is seen in *Fucus vesiculosus*, a marine alga (Bhowmick et al., 2020; Catarino et al., 2018). This alga contains oligomeric phlorotannins that consist of three to eight structural units of phloroglucinol, which is a polyphenol that exerts significant antimicrobial activity against several strains of Gram-positive bacteria including *S. aureus* and *Streptococcus pneumoniae* (Bhowmick et al., 2020; Mittal et al., 2019; National Center for Biotechnology Information, 2021).

Another polyphenol commonly found in algae is bromophenol (Bhowmick et al., 2020). Bromophenols are also made up of phenols, except that these phenols have bromine atoms attached to the phenol backbone (Bhowmick et al., 2020). Just like the other typical polyphenols extracted from algae, bromophenols possess properties associated with medicine, like anticancer, antidiabetic, antimicrobial, and anti-inflammatory activities (Bhowmick et al., 2020). A previous study has investigated the bioactivities of four bromophenols from a marine red alga, *Rhodomela confervoides*, and revealed their potent antibacterial activities against *S. aureus* and *P. aeruginosa* (Lijun et al., 2005). Another more recent study shows that these marine algal bromophenols extracted from a marine red alga named *Kappaphycus alvarezii*, can be modified with benzene, methyl, and glycosyl substitutions (Cherian et al., 2019). These modified bromophenols would then express improved ability to inhibit bacteria, stability, and pharmacokinetic properties (Cherian et al., 2019). Specifically, they were shown to be able to effectively inhibit a gram-negative bacterium, *Porphyromonas gingivalis* (*P. gingivalis*), which is able to resist *in vitro* antibiotic treatment

(Cherian et al., 2019; Irshad et al., 2012). These modified bromophenols are able to control the growth of *P. gingivalis*, and it is hypothesized that this is achieved through inhibition of the bacterial proteins' activity and production at both the protein and gene level (Cherian et al., 2019; Irshad et al., 2012). This, again, proves that algae holds great potential and value in the field of drug discovery.

## Fatty Acids from Algae

Fatty acids are carboxylic acids with long carbon chains (McKee et al., 2020). Most life forms depend on fatty acids to form and maintain the integrity of membranes and cellular organization (Bhowmick et al., 2020). It has been observed that fatty acids tend to get released by the algal cells when they lose integrity, and it is hypothesized that this is a defence mechanism employed when the cells are under attack by pathogenic bacteria and predators (Bhowmick et al., 2020). It has also been pointed out that the antibacterial potency of these free fatty acids correlates with the level of unsaturation and length of the carbon chains: the longer and more unsaturated the carbon chain, the greater its antibacterial activity (Bhowmick et al., 2020; Kabara et al., 1972).

A number of mechanisms have been proposed for how free fatty acids carry out their antibacterial activities, but it is said the prime targets are likely the bacterial cell membrane and the essential processes that take place at or within the membrane (Desbois and Smith, 2010). As these free fatty acids are amphipathic in nature, they are able to act as detergents by interacting with the cell membrane and creating transient or permanent pores of variable sizes (Desbois and Smith, 2010). At higher concentrations, they can even solubilize the membrane to an extent where membrane proteins or larger sections of the lipid bilayer get released (Desbois and Smith, 2010). Moreover, they can interfere with the activity of the electron transport chain (ETC) and disrupt oxidative phosphorylation, thereby affecting the energy supply of the bacterial cells (Desbois and Smith, 2010). There are a variety of other processes which they can impact to inhibit the growth of or kill the bacterial cells, some are cell lysis, enzyme inhibition, impairment of nutrient uptake, and generation of toxic peroxidation and autoxidation products (Desbois and Smith, 2010).

On the other hand, there are bacteria species that are naturally resistant to the antibacterial actions of these free fatty acids (Desbois and Smith, 2010). This is due to the fact that some bacterial species are able to manipulate their cell surface hydrophobicity, which can affect the free fatty acids' ability to permeate the outer membrane or cell wall, and block their access to their target sites on the inner membrane (Desbois and Smith, 2010). For instance, *S. aureus* can upregulate the synthesis of proteins involved in building the cell walls upon exposure to unsaturated free fatty acids, create a thicker cell wall and increase the difficulty of penetration by the fatty acids (Desbois and Smith, 2010). However, this does not imply that the free fatty acids have less value in medicine. They are abundant in nature, generally non-toxic and safe to use, so they are still considered attractive antibacterial agents, especially in scenarios where the use of conventional antibiotics may be undesirable

(Desbois and Smith, 2010).

One example of the antibacterial activity exerted by free algal fatty acids can be seen with *Scenedesmus obliquus*, a green algae species (Bhowmick et al., 2020; Afify et al., 2018). The long chain fatty acids isolated from this species can inhibit pathogenic bacteria like *S. aureus*, *E. coli*, and *P. aeruginosa* (Bhowmick et al., 2020). Another example is the red algae species, *Gracilaria edulis*, which has fatty acid extracts that can inhibit the bacteria *Aeromona hydrophila* (*A. hydrophila*) (Bhowmick et al., 2020). As previously mentioned, there are bacteria that can thicken their cell walls and become resistant to these fatty acids' action, but a lot of different bacteria strains still remain susceptible to them (Bhowmick et al., 2020). Hence, fatty acids, like the other extracts from algae, have the potential of being used as an alternative to conventional antibiotics (Bhowmick et al., 2020).

## Pigments from Algae

Pigments are what give the algae their colour, which has allowed for their classification into three main classes stated above (brown algae, red algae, and green algae) (Pérez et al., 2016). Algae can produce pigments because of their photosynthetic nature (Pérez et al., 2016). The following are the major pigments present in algae: fucoxanthin, chlorophylls a and c, are responsible for the brown colour; phycobilins for the red colour; and chlorophylls a and b for the green colour (Pérez et al., 2016). These pigments serve different functions in algae, some are central components for photosynthesis, and some make the algae photoprotective, protecting them from damage by sunlight (Pérez et al., 2016).

Similar to the other algal extracts introduced, algal pigments exert antibacterial activity (Silva et al., 2020; Pérez et al., 2016). For instance, fucoxanthin extracted from the brown alga *Himanthalia elongata* (*H. elongata*) can inhibit the bacteria *Listeria monocytogenes* (*L. monocytogenes*) (Silva et al., 2020; Rajauria and Abu-Ghannam, 2013). The proposed mechanism states that the pigments can increase permeability of the bacterial cell membranes, cause leakage of the cytoplasm, and also inhibit nucleic acid formation (Silva et al., 2020). Note that their mechanism of action has not been fully elucidated and more research is required (Silva et al., 2020).

## Conclusion

As the crisis of antibiotics resistance escalates, different sources of compounds or natural products are being explored for their potential to become antibacterial agents. Among the many compounds or substances found in nature, algae are definitely one of the most appealing sources. There is a variety of algae species living in complex habitats, which encourage evolution of the metabolites, leading to antibacterial properties that can be harnessed and be used to develop novel antibiotics. Algae are also attractive due to their accessibility and abundance in nature, as well as their non-toxicity. It is hopeful that in the near future, with more in-depth research, algae can become a reliable source of antibacterial agents, contributing to not only drug discovery, but also the development of other biomedical applications.

# Chapter 10: Confronting Antibiotic Resistance beyond the COVID-19 pandemic
## Future Perspectives and What to Consider Moving Forward

By: Dr. Austin Mardon & Suad Alad

## Introduction

With modern society beginning to shift and change socially due to the presence and effects of the COVID-19 pandemic, many questions, thoughts and concerns arise regarding what will occur in the future: What does a post-COVID world look like? How will we navigate through it? Will practices we've adopted become abandoned as we begin to return to normal, whatever that normal entails, or will we bring them along with us moving forward? How will medical procedures and protocols change as we move forward? *What* is there to *expect*? *What* should we *consider*?

Reading this very text has provided readers with a plethora of information regarding antibiotic resistance throughout history, therapies and remedies to combat these forms of mutation and how in the midst of COVID-19, the way antibiotic resistance has increased during its presence. As society begins to approach a world foreign to the one of our contemporary and past understanding, it is important to have these conversations and questions in mind.

Throughout this final chapter, these questions will be both asked and answered, and a conversation regarding a future beyond the COVID-19 pandemic will be brought forth. The purpose of said conversation is to bring awareness to past perspectives that may have not been considered at the start of the pandemic and to present possible solutions for what is to come if these same issues arise in the future both regarding antibiotic resistance and the socioeconomic factors that surround it.

## Bacterial Infections, Antibiotic Stewardship and Its Contribution to the Resistance Spike

Studies have shown that throughout the course of the COVID-19 pandemic there has been an influx of antibiotic resistance present in those infected by the virus at the pandemic's start. This was a result of symptoms regarding COVID-19 being unclear to the general public and those experiencing symptoms due to the overuse or misuse of antibiotics to try to cure or subside these symptoms. According to the Harvard Graduate School of Arts and Science approximately 70-79% of those hospitalized with

COVID-19 were treated with antibiotic therapy, despite the fact that COVID-19 is a virus, not a bacterial infection and cannot be cured or treated through the use of antibiotics.

This usage was only increased in patients with low function immune systems who ran the risk of exposure to secondary infections (bacterial and fungal) being in such close proximity with various forms of illness that could have been critical to said patients (Sagren, 2021). This usage was both precaution and medical protocol and at the time, appeared as the only way to rapidly treat and prevent whatever illness that may present itself within these patients. Prior to the pandemic the use of antibiotics was used in moments of necessity, typically only used when found to be absolutely necessary (McKenna, 2020). However, throughout COVID-19's start, patients experiencing extreme cases of the virus' symptoms became susceptible to these very secondary bacterial and fungal infections, received high dosage of antibiotics and began resisting the medication being administered (McKenna 2020).

According to a study conducted in Wuhan, China, 191 patients recorded between two hospitals received secondary bacterial infections within 15% of those admitted with COVID-19, and of those 15%, 7.5% of them died (Zhouct al., 2020). Prior to the pandemic, physicians within the medical community followed what is widely known as antibiotic or antimicrobial stewardship, which is the medical practice of using antibiotic medication consciously to avoid the curation of organisms that will mutate into become resistant to said antibiotics (Public Health Ontario 2019).

Maryn McKenna, contributor for *WIRED Science*, writes "[a] key principle of [antibiotic] stewardship is making sure that the infections a patient is experiencing are identified and lab-confirmed [...] / It is not routine practice to give antibiotics simply because someone has been placed on a ventilator. But in COVID-19 care, diagnostic procedures that would justify antibiotics—such as snaking a tube into the lungs for a visual exam or retrieving samples of lung fluid—expose health care workers to too much risk" (McKenna, 2020). This form of exposure only increased the administration of the drugs, and when the dosage administered did not do an adequate job, the dosages were increased, and thus created a vicious cycle of antibiotic use. Usage of antibiotics had become so high that multiple antibiotic manufacturers had district wide shortages; something unheard of prior to the pandemic's start.

Clearly, there is an issue regarding antibiotic administration that is not being addressed. In her article, McKenna (2020) makes it clear that it is not anyone's desire to cut off the usage or prescription of antibiotics, but rather what is needed is a sense of consciousness that must be made aware to both the medical community as well as the general public. Other options must be considered, preached and practiced in replacement of mass purchasing and misusing antibiotics to treat illnesses that are not treatable or require antibiotics in the first place.

So what needs to happen as time goes on? How and why can the presentation of antibiotic resistance begin to dwindle? What needs to be done and how can it continue to be done in the future? With COVID-19's presence within the last year and a half, the concept of illness has definitely changed. With that change, has come what many have described as a hyper-consciousness of hygiene and cleanliness. This hyper-consciousness, although fairly new, has been recorded as a step in the right direction regarding this shift in our relationship with illness and medication (Sagren, 2021). What is needed is a shift in one's understanding of illness, how to treat it and essentially how to prevent it so the necessity of drug use is seen as an unnecessary option. In a hyper-conscious world of hygiene, prevention of viral spread is caught early on and the necessity of antibiotic use is decreased (Sagren, 2021).

## How Hyper-conscious Hygiene Stunted Antibiotic Use and Resistance

What has been found as the pandemic has continued is that while antibiotic treatment has been high, the consciousness of hygiene, personal space and isolation during times of illness has become extremely prevalent within our culture and could very well be how rates of antibiotic resistance can decrease in future's time (Minnesota Department of Health, 2019). As previously stated, there was a large influx regarding the use of antibiotics when treating COVID-19 or COVID-19 related symptoms. And thus, increased the potential for antibiotic resistance within patients. However, some studies have found as the pandemic continues on, our current habits regarding hygiene and health have become extremely hyperconscious. As reference above, antibiotics cannot cure viral infections and their purpose is to treat bacterial infections. However, handwashing kills and prevents the spread of germs between physical contact and can be a crucial practice in the prevention of bacterial transition (Minnesota Department of Health, 2019). Viral infections consist of illness such as the flu, the common cold, bronchitis etc. They require a host for transmission (Davis, 2020). Bacterial infections differ from viral infections because unlike viral infections, bacterial infections do not require a host for reproduction (Davis, 2020).

Promotion of hygiene and cleanliness as a means to both prevent COVID-19 as well as keep those around one another safe has made our way into mainstream aspects of our everyday lives; in street signs, televised commercials, online ads, through the form of subscription information (being emailed COVID-19 safety tips' along with typical subscription information), etc. People in the current, and potentially once it arrives, post COVID-19 world have been taking extreme steps towards being generally more hygenic at more frequent rates than in year's past. In a survey conducted of 1000 participants by Henkel Canada (an Adhesive Technology, Home and Beauty Care Company] for Dial Soap Canada regarding Canadian hygiene practices in the current COVID-19 world, it was found that the average Canadian only washed their hands approximately 3-4 times in one day.

Since the pandemic's start and during its succession, this number has tripled in action, with the average Canadian now washing their hands about 10-11 times a day. A third of those participating within the survey said they only washed their hands before eating "sometimes" and that prior to the pandemic of 90%, only 48.6% washed their hands for the recommended 20 seconds. With this data alone, it has been proven that the awareness of germs and its contraction through touch has increased greatly and that

Canadians [and assumably others across the globe] have become hyper-conscious of not only how important hand washing is in the safety and health of one another, but also how prevalent it is in preventing and combating illness and bacterial disease.

In the same article with the Harvard Graduate School of Arts and Science referenced earlier in this chapter, it states one of the best ways to prevent infectious disease and virus is the very practice of personal and social hygiene. This would entail, washing one's hands on a regular basis, especially in situations where germs or other bacteria are prominent through touch are extremely plausible. And with the presence of the COVID-19 pandemic, this practice has not only been amplified, but as a plausible outcome of getting this disease is death, people's consciousness only grows stronger. In a present COVID-19 world, it is highly unlikely to see someone not wash their hands continuously throughout a day and if soap and water is not accessible at the moment in time, the use of hand sanitizer has become all the more prominent. Paired with the practices of social distancing, restricting close contact to those most necessary in one's life [as hard as it may be to decipher and decide who that may be], the prevalence of personal and social hygienics became a large factor in preventing the spread of the virus. And as these practices become adopted within our culture as the new normal 'standards' of hygiene, the prevention of COVID-19, and other potential viruses only becomes more prominent.

Unfortunately, however, this course of action is not enough to terminate the pandemic's stay within the modern world. And for some, it is not exactly an action that is plausible to everyone.

Especially those who are experiencing restriction of access to these important resources that can prevent the spread of the virus in the first place. This consideration and perspective brings about the question of who and why; the answers being those in low income communities and for the reason that their socioeconomic status prevents them from accessing the sanitization products needed to prevent the virus.

## Low Income Access to Sanitary Equipment and How The Negligence of Their Perspective Has Hurt Reaching the Pandemic's End

It is no secret that those existing within poverty or lower income groups and communities have been a part of a group whose experiences, necessities and perspectives have been both neglected and ignored. Previous to the pandemic and COVID-19's existence, those within poverty have been left to fend for themselves in situations regarding health care, access to water, food security and employment. So, as unfortunate as it may appear, it is no surprise that they have become a perspective that has failed to be considered thus far. However, what is most concerning about this negligence is the rate in which low income communities have presented themselves within statistics regarding contractions of the virus, as well as deaths of the virus.

It has been recorded by the Canadian Government that the communities hit the worst with COVID-19 and the communities with the highest mortality rate with COVID-19 being the primary cause have been communities that are highly racialized and by extension make up the population of the country that are relatively poor or financially insecure (Government of Canada, 2020). According to these statistics, within Montreal and Toronto respectively, these two cities within Canada recorded having the highest population deaths of COVID-19.

In Montreal, the South Asian population made up the majority percentage of these deaths, and in Toronto, Black Canadians made up its majority. As of 2019, South Asian's living in Canada makeup 16.5% of citizens living in relatively low income communities and Black Canadians 23.8% (Government of Canada, 2019). These statistics cannot be considered a coincidence. These rates illustrate at what disproportion those living within these communities are affected by lack of sanitization products, masks, opportunities for social distancing and possibilities for self isolation and sick leave *if* necessary. And because a majority of these practices [excluding paid sick leaves and self isolation periods] have become such normalized adoptions within our contemporary world, those who cannot adopt these very practices are essentially excluded or left behind. This may propose the question: Why are these people being excluded?

At the pandemic's start, countries with infrastructures that are globally considered 'weaker' or 'lower' that modes of Westernization were put into positions of desperation and ultimately left defenceless against the virus (Mills, 2020). Relatively, these same concerns and feelings can be extended to those living within similar economic statuses within these same Western countries. An unfortunate fact is that access to something as simple as clean water is not a reality for billions living in the world and of those billions, millions live within the West. 74% of First Nations citizens living in Canada face advisories accessing clean water (Bui, 2020). Without access to this clean water, the opportunity to wash one's hands is left a scarce option and when one *does* access clean water, they are left making the choice to drink it, bathe in it or clean with it, and usually this form of cleaning is not used on handwashing (Mills, 2020). As Mills states in his article, perspectives of what is required for someone differs between income classes. Someone of a middle or higher income class' main concerns at the start of the pandemic were who would be "[disinfecting their] groceries" (Mills, 2020) while those living in situations of poverty or low income wondered where they would be getting their next meal or if they would still be keeping their jobs; and as previously stated, where they would be finding water. Where does this leave them in a present COVID-19 world, where access to clean water is crucial in the prevention of virus spreading? Well, it leaves them in a position of vulnerability, exposure to a virus that has a high statistical rate of killing them (Government of Canada, 2020) or leaving them ill for extended periods of time.

## What Now?: The One Health Approach and Next Steps For the Future

So where does this lead to? What is to be done with this information? What needs to be expected or considered for the future? What should continue to be done? In relation to the previous argument regarding low income communities and the spread of COVID-19 throughout these groups is necessary in the acknowledgement of preventing the overall spread of the virus in general, an important aspect of this argument is the strength in community building and solidarity. When people come together to solve an issue or come up with plans to prevent future tragedy or hardship, the plausibility of creating solutions of universal access and equitability are far greater to achieve. A solution found within medical sciences that also adopts principles of philosophy and social justice is the 'One Health Approach'.

The One Health Approach is what the Center for Disease Control (CDC) describes as a transdisciplinary practice "with the goal of achieving optimal health outcomes recognizing the interconnection between people, animals, plants, and their shared environment" (CDC, 2018). Essentially this social practice asks those participating in it to reflect on their own impacts within the environment, those living in it and how everyone's health, including animals, are interconnected within one another. A sense of community is highly emphasized and collaboration amongst different groups and consideration of one another is encouraged.

The way the One Health Approach is meant to operate is incorporating professionals in human, animal and environmental health into the structures of prosaic communities to curate activities and social projects to improve the benefit of multitude sectors of health. This approach's focus on solving the issue of privileged communities neglecting perspectives outside of one another's own personal experiences and provides communities that are typically left without access to professional advice or guidance direct interaction with these professionals. The CDC states on their website that with the One Health Approach, society "can achieve the best health outcomes for people, animals, and plants in a shared environment" (CDC, 2018).

With this approach in mind and underway, as it is not a new method, community building, as well as social, political and economic issues are addressed and practices towards universal health are implemented. In regards to antibiotic resistance, a better standard of health and an improved structure of hygiene and illness prevention can further prevent the infections that require antibiotic treatment. Through this form precaution and collaboration education on how illness spreads between humans, animals and plants is provided and thus illness across the margins has a lower plausibility for spread (CDC, 2018). Which, in turn, limits the exposure of infection, the overuse of antibiotics and the potential for antibiotic resistance.

## Conclusion

The end of COVID-19 is one that unfortunately does not have a set date or time attached to it. With each passing day, new information is presented to the public and different methodologies and practices become integrated within the contemporary times and the world begins to adopt what is known as the new normal. However, with this presentation of the new normal and essentially a new world, the information known prior to this foreign environment is just as valuable as the information succeeding it.

COVID-19 has reaffirmed the necessity in considering the genuinely pressing issue regarding the misuse of antibiotics and how this misuse has increased the spike within its resistance and has asked the world to step and consider everyday issues throughout the world beyond COVID-19. As society moves forward to a world beyond the COVID-19 pandemic, consideration of these issues, these perspectives and the solutions that follow are essential in curating a world of health, freedom, safety and ensuring that in moments of desperation, society is leaning amongst one another instead of turning against one another.

# References

## *Chapter 1:*

CDC. (2014). *Antibiotic prescribing and use in doctor's offices: Measuring outpatient antibiotic prescribing.* https://www.cdc.gov/antibiotic-use/community/programs-measurement/measuring-antibiotic-prescribing.html

CDC. (2016). *Tuberculosis (TB): Basic TB facts.* https://www.cdc.gov/tb/topic/basics/default.htm

CDC. (2017). *Sexually transmitted diseases (STDs): Basic fact sheet.* https://www.cdc.gov/std/syphilis/stdfact-syphilis.htm

CDC. (2020). *Typhus fevers: Epidemic typhus.* https://www.cdc.gov/typhus/epidemic/index.html

Chopra, I., & Roberts, M. (2001). Tetracycline antibiotics: mode of action, applications, molecular biology, and epidemiology of bacterial resistance. *Microbiology and molecular biology reviews : MMBR, 65*(2), 232–260. https://doi.org/10.1128/MMBR.65.2.232-260.2001

Davies, J. (2006). Where have all the antibiotics gone? *Can J Infect Dis Med Microbiol*, 17(5): 287–290. https://doi.org/10.1155/2006/707296

Demain A. L. (2009). Antibiotics: natural products essential to human health. *Medicinal research reviews*, 29(6), 821–842. https://doi.org/10.1002/med.20154

Durand, G. A., Raoult, D., Dubourg, G. (2019). Antibiotic

discovery: history, methods and perspectives. *International Journal of Antimicrobial Agents,* 53(4), 371-382. https://doi.org/ 10.1016/j.ijantimicag.2018.11.010

Farzam, K., Nessel, T. A , & Quick, J. (2020) Erythromycin. *StatPearls [Internet].* https://www.ncbi.nlm.nih.gov/books/ NBK532249/

Fleming A. (1929) On the antibacterial action of cultures of a penicillium, with special reference to their use in the isolation of B. influenzae. *British Journal of Experimental Pathology*, 10, 226-236.

Genilloud, O. (2017). Actinomycetes: still a source of novel antibiotics. *Nat. Prod. Rep.,* 34, 1203-1232. https://doi.org/ 10.1039/C7NP00026J

Germovsek, E., Barker, C. I., & Sharland, M. (2017). What do I need to know about aminoglycoside antibiotics?. *Arc. Dis. Child Edu. Pract. Ed.*, *102*(2), 89–93. https://doi.org/10.1136/ archdischild-2015-309069

Gould, K. (2016). Antibiotics: from prehistory to the present day. *Journal of Antimicrobial Chemotherapy,* 71(3), 572-575. https:// doi.org/10.1093/jac/dkv484

Government of Canada. (2019). *Antibiotic use in Canada: Preserving antibiotics now and in the future.* https:// www.canada.ca/en/public-health/corporate/publications/chief-public-health-officer-reports-state-public-health-canada/ preserving-antibiotics/antibiotic-use.html

Hutchings, M. I., Truman A. W., & Wilkinson, B. (2019).
Antibiotics: past, present and future. *Current Opinion in
Microbiology,* 51, 72-80. https://doi.org/10.1016/
j.mib.2019.10.008

Microbiology Society. (2015). *The history of antibiotics.* https://
microbiologysociety.org/members-outreach-resources/outreach-
resources/antibiotics-unearthed/antibiotics-and-antibiotic-
resistance/the-history-of-antibiotics.html

Mohr, K. I. (2016). History of antibiotics research. *Current
Topics in Microbiology and Immunology,* 398, 237-272. https://
doi.org/10.1007/82_2016_499

National Cancer Institute. (n.d.). *NCI Dictionary of Cancer
Terms.* https://www.cancer.gov/publications/dictionaries/cancer-
terms/def/microorganism

National Institutes of Health. (2012). *How sulfa drugs work.*
https://www.nih.gov/news-events/nih-research-matters/how-
sulfa-drugs-work

NHS. (2018a). *Azithromycin.* https://www.nhs.uk/medicines/
azithromycin/

NHS. (2018b). *Chloramphenicol.* https://www.nhs.uk/medicines/
chloramphenicol/

NHS. (2018c). *Doxycycline.* https://www.nhs.uk/medicines/
doxycycline/

Nicolaou, K. & Rigol, S. (2018). A brief history of antibiotics and select advances in their synthesis. *J Antibiot,* 71, 153-184. https://doi.org/10.1038/ja.2017.62

OED Online. (2021). Antibiotic, adj. and n. *Oxford University Press. https://www.oed.com/view/Entry/8513? redirectedFrom=antibiotics*

Ribeiro da Cunha, B., Fonseca, L. P., & Calado, C. R. C. (2019). Antibiotic discovery: Where have we come from, where do we go? *Antibiotics,* 8(2), 45. https://doi.org/10.3390/ antibiotics8020045

Silhavy, T. J., Kahne, D., & Walker, S. (2010). The bacterial cell envelope. *Cold Spring Harbor perspectives in biology*, 2(5), a000414. https://doi.org/10.1101/cshperspect.a000414

The Nobel Prize. (2021). *All Nobel Prizes in physiology and medicine.* https://www.nobelprize.org/prizes/lists/all-nobel-laureates-in-physiology-or-medicine/

U.S. National Library of Medicine. (2016). *Vancomycin. https:// medlineplus.gov/druginfo/meds/a604038.html*

U.S. National Library of Medicine. (2021). *Penicillin v potassium.* https://medlineplus.gov/druginfo/meds/a685015.html

Waksman, S. A. (1947). What is an antibiotic or an antibiotic substance?. *Mycologia*, 39(5), 565–569.

Weber, T., Charusanti, P., Musiol-Kroll, E. M., Jiang, X., Tong, Y., Kim, H. U., & Lee, S. Y. (2015). Metabolic engineering of antibiotic factories: new tools for antibiotic production in actinomycetes. *Trends in Biotechnology,* 33(1), 15-26. https://doi.org/10.1016/j.tibtech.2014.10.009

## *Chapter 2:*

Abraham, E. P., & Chain, E. (1940). An Enzyme from Bacteria able to Destroy Penicillin. Nature, 146(3713), 837–837. https://doi.org/10.1038/146837a0

Beardmore, R. E., Peña-Miller, R., Gori, F., & Iredell, J. (2017). Antibiotic Cycling and Antibiotic Mixing: Which One Best Mitigates Antibiotic Resistance? Molecular Biology and Evolution, 34(4), 802–817. https://doi.org/10.1093/molbev/msw292

CDC. (2020, March 13). What Exactly is Antibiotic Resistance? Centers for Disease Control and Prevention. https://www.cdc.gov/drugresistance/about.html

Dall, C. (2016, December 22). FDA: Antibiotic use in food animals continues to rise. CIDRAP. https://www.cidrap.umn.edu/news-perspective/2016/12/fda-antibiotic-use-food-animals-continues-rise

Dall, C. (2018, January 26). Antibiotic cycling, mixing don't affect resistance, study says. CIDRAP. https://www.cidrap.umn.edu/news-perspective/2018/01/antibiotic-cycling-mixing-dont-affect-resistance-study-says

Davies, J., & Davies, D. (2010). Origins and Evolution of

Antibiotic Resistance. Microbiology and Molecular Biology Reviews, 74(3), 417–433. https://doi.org/10.1128/MMBR.00016-10

Foster, T. J. (2017). Antibiotic resistance in Staphylococcus aureus. Current status and future prospects. FEMS Microbiology Reviews, 41(3), 430–449. https://doi.org/10.1093/femsre/fux007

Gould, K. (2016). Antibiotics: From prehistory to the present day. Journal of Antimicrobial Chemotherapy, 71(3), 572–575. https://doi.org/10.1093/jac/dkv484

Luyt, C.-E., Bréchot, N., Trouillet, J.-L., & Chastre, J. (2014). Antibiotic stewardship in the intensive care unit. Critical Care, 18(5). https://doi.org/10.1186/s13054-014-0480-6

Manyi-Loh, C., Mamphweli, S., Meyer, E., & Okoh, A. (2018). Antibiotic Use in Agriculture and Its Consequential Resistance in Environmental Sources: Potential Public Health Implications. Molecules : A Journal of Synthetic Chemistry and Natural Product Chemistry, 23(4). https://doi.org/10.3390/molecules23040795

Shambaugh, G. E., JR. (1966). History of Sulfonamides. Archives of Otolaryngology, 83(1), 1–2. https://doi.org/10.1001/archotol.1966.00760020003001

Thomas, C., & Nielsen, K. (2005). Thomas CM, Nielsen KM. Mechanisms of, and barriers to, horizontal gene transfer between bacteria. Nat Rev Micro 3: 711-721. Nature Reviews. Microbiology, 3, 711–721. https://doi.org/10.1038/nrmicro1234

Ventola, C. L. (2015). The Antibiotic Resistance Crisis.
Pharmacy and Therapeutics, 40(4), 277–283.

Walsh, C., & Wencewicz, T. (2016). Antibiotics: Challenges,
Mechanisms, Opportunities. John Wiley & Sons.

Wencewicz, T. A., & Miller, M. J. (2018). Sideromycins as
Pathogen-Targeted Antibiotics. In J. F. Fisher, S. Mobashery, &
M. J. Miller (Eds.), Antibacterials: Volume II (pp. 151–183).
Springer International Publishing. https://doi.org/
10.1007/7355_2017_19

WHO. (2019). World Health Organization Model List of
Essential Medicines. https://www.who.int/publications-detail-
redirect/WHOMVPEMPIAU2019.06

WHO. (2020, October 13). Antimicrobial resistance. World
Health Organization. https://www.who.int/en/news-room/fact-
sheets/detail/antimicrobial-resistance

Wright, G. D. (2012). The origins of antibiotic resistance.
Handbook of Experimental Pharmacology, 211, 13–30. https://
doi.org/10.1007/978-3-642-28951-4_2

## Chapter 3:

Abou Dagher, G., El Khuri, C., Chehadeh, A. A.-H., Chami, A.,
Bachir, R., Zebian, D., & Bou Chebl, R. (2017). Are patients
with cancer with sepsis and bacteraemia at a higher risk of
mortality? A retrospective chart review of patients presenting to

a tertiary care centre in Lebanon. *BMJ Open*, *7*(3). https://doi.org/10.1136/bmjopen-2016-013502

Adedeji W. A. (2016). THE TREASURE CALLED ANTIBIOTICS. Annals of Ibadan postgraduate medicine, 14(2), 56–57

Alamrew, K., Tadesse, T. A., Abiye, A. A., & Shibeshi, W. (2019). Surgical Antimicrobial Prophylaxis and Incidence of Surgical Site Infections at Ethiopian Tertiary-Care Teaching Hospital. *Infectious Diseases: Research and Treatment*, *12*, 117863371989226. https://doi.org/10.1177/1178633719892267

Andersen, B. M. (2018). Prevention of Postoperative Wound Infections. *Prevention and Control of Infections in Hospitals*, 377–437. https://doi.org/10.1007/978-3-319-99921-0_33

Arruebo, M., Vilaboa, N., Sáez-Gutiérrez, B., Lambea, J., Tres, A., Valladares, M., & González-Fernández, Á. (2011). Assessment of the Evolution of Cancer Treatment Therapies. *Cancers*, *3*(3), 3279–3330. https://doi.org/10.3390/cancers3033279

Baue, A. E. (1998). The Complexities of Sepsis and Organ Dysfunction. *Sepsis and Organ Dysfunction*, 23–31. https://doi.org/10.1007/978-88-470-2271-3_2

Bernell, S., & Howard, S. W. (2016). Use Your Words Carefully: What Is a Chronic Disease? *Frontiers in Public Health*, *4*, 159. https://doi.org/10.3389/fpubh.2016.00159

Carney, E. F. (2020). The impact of chronic kidney disease on global health. *Nature Reviews Nephrology*, *16*(5), 251–251. https://doi.org/10.1038/s41581-020-0268-7

Centers for Disease Control and Prevention. (2020, December 7). *Clinical Information*. Centers for Disease Control and Prevention. https://www.cdc.gov/sepsis/clinicaltools/ index.html#:~:text=Each%20year%2C%20at%20least%201.7,in %20a%20hospital%20has%20sepsis

Centers for Disease Control and Prevention. (2020, February 7). *Chronic Kidney Disease Basics*. Centers for Disease Control and Prevention. https://www.cdc.gov/kidneydisease/basics.html

Chang, C.-H., Fan, P.-C., Kuo, G., Lin, Y.-S., Tsai, T.-Y., Chang, S.-W., … Lee, C.-C. (2020). Infection in Advanced Chronic Kidney Disease and Subsequent Adverse Outcomes after Dialysis Initiation: A Nationwide Cohort Study. *Scientific Reports*, *10*(1). https://doi.org/10.1038/s41598-020-59794-7

Chavers, B. M., Solid, C. A., Gilbertson, D. T., & Collins, A. J. (2007). Infection-Related Hospitalization Rates in Pediatric versus Adult Patients with End-Stage Renal Disease in the United States. *Journal of the American Society of Nephrology*, *18*(3), 952–959. https://doi.org/10.1681/asn.2006040406

Cornejo-Juárez, P., Vilar-Compte, D., Pérez-Jiménez, C., Ñamendys-Silva, S. A., Sandoval-Hernández, S., & Volkow-Fernández, P. (2015). The impact of hospital-acquired infections with multidrug-resistant bacteria in an oncology intensive care unit. *International Journal of Infectious Diseases*, *31*, 31–34.

https://doi.org/10.1016/j.ijid.2014.12.022

Crader MF, Varacallo M. (2021) Preoperative Antibiotic Prophylaxis. *StatPearls*.

Critchley, J. A., Carey, I. M., Harris, T., DeWilde, S., Hosking, F. J., & Cook, D. G. (2018). Glycemic Control and Risk of Infections Among People With Type 1 or Type 2 Diabetes in a Large Primary Care Cohort Study. *Diabetes Care*, *41*(10), 2127–2135. https://doi.org/10.2337/dc18-0287

Dalrymple, L. S., & Go, A. S. (2008). Epidemiology of Acute Infections among Patients with Chronic Kidney Disease: Figure 1. *Clinical Journal of the American Society of Nephrology*, *3*(5), 1487–1493. https://doi.org/10.2215/cjn.01290308

De Simone, B., Sartelli, M., Coccolini, F., Ball, C. G., Brambillasca, P., Chiarugi, M., … Catena, F. (2020). Intraoperative surgical site infection control and prevention: a position paper and future addendum to WSES intra-abdominal infections guidelines. *World Journal of Emergency Surgery*, *15*(1). https://doi.org/10.1186/s13017-020-0288-4

Duncan, M. D. (2005). Transplant-related Immunosuppression: A Review of Immunosuppression and Pulmonary Infections. *Proceedings of the American Thoracic Society*, *2*(5), 449–455. https://doi.org/10.1513/pats.200507-073js

Hotchkiss, R. S., Moldawer, L. L., Opal, S. M., Reinhart, K., Turnbull, I. R., & Vincent, J.-L. (2016). Sepsis and septic shock. *Nature Reviews Disease Primers*, *2*(1). https://doi.org/10.1038/

nrdp.2016.45

Huttunen, R., & Syrjänen, J. (2012). Obesity and the risk and outcome of infection. *International Journal of Obesity*, *37*(3), 333–340. https://doi.org/10.1038/ijo.2012.62

Jiang, Y., Dou, X., Yan, C., Wan, L., Liu, H., Li, M., … Wan, K. (2020). Epidemiological characteristics and trends of notifiable infectious diseases in China from 1986 to 2016. *Journal of Global Health*, *10*(2). https://doi.org/10.7189/jogh.10.020803

Meara, J. G., & Greenberg, S. L. M. (2015). Global Surgery Global surgery 2030: Evidence and solutions for achieving health, welfare and economic development. *The Lancet*, *386*(5), 834–835. https://doi.org/10.1016/j.surg.2015.02.009

Nesher, L., & Rolston, K. V. (2013). The current spectrum of infection in cancer patients with chemotherapy related neutropenia. *Infection*, *42*(1), 5–13. https://doi.org/10.1007/s15010-013-0525-9

Roser, M., Ortiz-Ospina, E., & Ritchie, H. (2019, October 23). *Life Expectancy*. Our World in Data. https://ourworldindata.org/life-expectancy#:~:text=The%20United%20Nations%20estimate%20a,life%20expectancy%20of%2072.3%20years

Rudd, K. E., Johnson, S. C., Agesa, K. M., Shackelford, K. A., Tsoi, D., Kievlan, D. R., … Naghavi, M. (2020). Global, regional, and national sepsis incidence and mortality, 1990–2017: analysis for the Global Burden of Disease Study. *The*

*Lancet*, *395*(10219), 200–211. https://doi.org/10.1016/s0140-6736(19)32989-7

Seung, K. J., Keshavjee, S., & Rich, M. L. (2015). Multidrug-Resistant Tuberculosis and Extensively Drug-Resistant Tuberculosis. Cold Spring Harbor Perspectives in Medicine, 5(9). https://doi.org/10.1101/cshperspect.a017863

Tan, S. Y., & Tatsumura, Y. (2015). Alexander Fleming (1881–1955): Discoverer of penicillin. *Singapore Medical Journal*, *56*(07), 366–367. https://doi.org/10.11622/smedj.2015105

Ventola C. L. (2015). The antibiotic resistance crisis: part 1: causes and threats. P & T : a peer-reviewed journal for formulary management, 40(4), 277–283.

Williams, M. D., Braun, L., Cooper, L. M., Johnston, J., Weiss, R. V., Qualy, R. L., & Linde-Zwirble, W. (2004). Hospitalized cancer patients with severe sepsis: analysis of incidence, mortality, and associated costs of care. *Critical Care*, *8*(5), 291–298. https://doi.org/10.1186/cc2893

Witter, A. R., Okunnu, B. M., & Berg, R. E. (2016). The Essential Role of Neutrophils during Infection with the Intracellular Bacterial PathogenListeria monocytogenes. *The Journal of Immunology*, *197*(5), 1557–1565. https://doi.org/10.4049/jimmunol.1600599

World Health Organization. (2020, October 13). *Antimicrobial resistance*. World Health Organization. https://www.who.int/news-room/fact-sheets/detail/antimicrobial-resistance

World Health Organization. (2021, March 3). *Cancer*. World Health Organization. https://www.who.int/news-room/fact-sheets/detail/cancer

World Health Organization. (n.d.). *Diabetes*. World Health Organization. https://www.who.int/health-topics/diabetes#tab=tab_1

World Health Organization. (2019, April 29). *New report calls for urgent action to avert antimicrobial resistance crisis*. World Health Organization. https://www.who.int/news/item/29-04-2019-new-report-calls-for-urgent-action-to-avert-antimicrobial-resistance-crisis

World Health Organization. (2020, April 1). *Obesity and overweight*. World Health Organization. https://www.who.int/news-room/fact-sheets/detail/obesity-and-overweight

World Health Organization. (2020, August 26). *Sepsis*. World Health Organization. https://www.who.int/news-room/fact-sheets/detail/sepsis

World Health Organization. (2020, December 9). *The top 10 causes of death*. World Health Organization. https://www.who.int/news-room/fact-sheets/detail/the-top-10-causes-of-death

World Health Organization. (2020, October 14). *Tuberculosis (TB)*. World Health Organization. https://www.who.int/news-room/fact-sheets/detail/tuberculosis#:~:text=Key%20facts,with%20tuberculosis(TB)

%20worldwide

World Health Organization. (2017, February 27). *WHO publishes list of bacteria for which new antibiotics are urgently needed*. World Health Organization. https://www.who.int/news/item/27-02-2017-who-publishes-list-of-bacteria-for-which-new-antibiotics-are-urgently-needed

World Health Organization. (2016, November 3). *WHO recommends 29 ways to stop surgical infections and avoid superbugs*. World Health Organization. https://www.who.int/news/item/03-11-2016-who-recommends-29-ways-to-stop-surgical-infections-and-avoid-superbugs


*Chapter 4:*

Reygaert, W.C (2018). An overview of the antimicrobial resistance mechanisms of bacteria. AIMS Microbiology, 4 (3), 482–501. https://doi.org/10.3934/microbiol.2018.3.482

Munita, J. M., & Arias, C. A. (2016). Mechanisms of Antibiotic Resistance. Microbiology Spectrum, 4 (2), 3–37. https://doi.org/10.1128/microbiolspec.vmbf-0016-2015

Reygaert, W. C. (2013, December 1). Antimicrobial resistance mechanisms of Staphylococcus aureus . ResearchGate. https://www.researchgate.net/publication/267695121_Antimicrobial_resistance_mechanisms_of_Staphylococcus_aureus

\* \* \*

## Chapter 5:

*Antibiotic resistance*. World Health Organization. (2020). Retrieved from https://www.who.int/news-room/fact-sheets/detail/antibiotic-resistance#:~:text=Antibiotic%20resistance%20leads%20to%20higher,will%20remain%20a%20major%20threat.

*Antibiotics - Side effects*. National Health Service. (2021). Retrieved from https://www.nhs.uk/conditions/antibiotics/side-effects/#:~:text=Antibiotic%20allergic%20reactions,coughing.

Boseley, S. (2020). *Big pharma failing to invest in new antibiotics, says WHO*. the Guardian. Retrieved from https://www.theguardian.com/business/2020/jan/17/big-pharma-failing-to-invest-in-new-antibiotics-says-who.

*Canadian Antimicrobial Resistance Surveillance System Report 2016* (2016). Canada.ca. Retrieved from https://www.canada.ca/en/public-health/services/publications/drugs-health-products/canadian-antimicrobial-resistance-surveillance-system-report-2016.html.

Choo, E. J., & Chambers, H. F. (2016). Treatment of methicillin-resistant Staphylococcus aureus bacteremia. *Infection & chemotherapy*, *48*(4), 267. Retrieved from https://www.ncbi.nlm.nih.gov/pmc/articles/PMC5204005/#:~:text=Vancomycin%20remains%20the%20initial%20antibiotic,alternative%2C%20and%20ceftaroline%20appears%20promisi ng.

Lee, C. (2008). Therapeutic challenges in the era of antibiotic resistance. International journal of antimicrobial agents, 32, S197-S199. Retrieved from https://pubmed.ncbi.nlm.nih.gov/19134519/

Liubakka, A., & Vaughn, B. P. (2016). Clostridium difficile infection and fecal microbiota transplant. *AACN advanced critical care*, *27*(3), 324-337. Retrieved from https://www.ncbi.nlm.nih.gov/pmc/articles/PMC5666691/

*NIH Human Microbiome Project defines normal bacterial makeup of the body*. National Institutes of Health (NIH). (2012). Retrieved from https://www.nih.gov/news-events/news-releases/nih-human-microbiome-project-defines-normal-bacterial-makeup-body#:~:text=This%20bacterial%20genomic%20contribution%20is,%E2%80%9D%20said%20Lita%20Proctor%2C%20Ph.

Nikaido, H. (2009). Multidrug resistance in bacteria. *Annual review of biochemistry*, *78*, 119-146. Retrieved from https://www.ncbi.nlm.nih.gov/pmc/articles/PMC2839888/#:~:text=More%20strains%20of%20pathogens%20have,of%20the%20commonly%20available%20agents.

Pichichero, M. E. (2006). Cephalosporins can be prescribed safely for penicillin-allergic patients. *Journal of family practice*, *55*(2), 106. Retrieved from https://pubmed.ncbi.nlm.nih.gov/16451776/#:~:text=The%20widely%20quoted%20cross%2Dallergy,among

%20patients%20with%20penicillin%20allergy.

Reizner, W., Hunter, J. G., O'Malley, N. T., Southgate, R. D., Schwarz, E. M., & Kates, S. L. (2014). A systematic review of animal models for Staphylococcus aureus osteomyelitis. *European cells & materials*, *27*, 196. Retrieved from https://www.ncbi.nlm.nih.gov/pmc/articles/PMC4322679/

Schmid, A., Wolfensberger, A., Nemeth, J., Schreiber, P. W., Sax, H., & Kuster, S. P. (2019). Monotherapy versus combination therapy for multidrug-resistant Gram-negative infections: Systematic Review and Meta-Analysis. *Scientific reports*, *9*(1), 1-11. Retrieved from https://www.nature.com/articles/s41598-019-51711-x

Tong, S. Y., Davis, J. S., Eichenberger, E., Holland, T. L., & Fowler, V. G. (2015). Staphylococcus aureus infections: epidemiology, pathophysiology, clinical manifestations, and management. *Clinical microbiology reviews*, *28*(3), 603-661. Retrieved from https://cmr.asm.org/content/28/3/603.short

*Tuberculosis (TB) - Treatment*. National Health Service. (2019). Retrieved from https://www.nhs.uk/conditions/tuberculosis-tb/treatment/#:~:text=You%27ll%20be%20prescribed%20at,and%20rifampicin.

Ventola, C. L. (2015). The antibiotic resistance crisis: part 1: causes and threats. *Pharmacy and therapeutics*, *40*(4), 277. Retrieved from https://www.ncbi.nlm.nih.gov/pmc/articles/

PMC4378521/

Why is it so hard to develop new antibiotics?. Wellcome. (2020). Retrieved from https://wellcome.org/news/why-is-it-so-hard-develop-new-antibiotics.

## *Chapter 6:*

Akova M. (2016). Epidemiology of antimicrobial resistance in bloodstream infections. *Virulence, 7*(3), 252–266. https://doi.org/10.1080/21505594.2016.1159366

Bawa, R., Bawa, S. R., Maebius, S. B., Flynn, T., & Wei, C. (2005). Protecting new ideas and inventions in nanomedicine with patents. *Nanomedicine: nanotechnology, biology, and medicine, 1*(2), 150–158. https://doi.org/10.1016/j.nano.2005.03.009

Center for Disease Control and Prevention (2021). How do germs become resistant? https://www.cdc.gov/drugresistance/about/how-resistance-happens.html

Donlan R. M. (2001). Biofilm formation: a clinically relevant microbiological process. *Clinical infectious diseases: an official publication of the Infectious Diseases Society of America, 33*(8), 1387–1392. https://doi.org/10.1086/322972

El-Sayed, A., & Kamel, M. (2020). Advances in nanomedical applications: diagnostic, therapeutic, immunization, and vaccine production. *Environmental science and pollution research international*, *27*(16), 19200–19213. https://doi.org/10.1007/s11356-019-06459-2

Eleraky, N.E., Allam, A., Hassan, S.B., & Omar, M.M. (2020). Nanomedicine Fight against Antibacterial Resistance: An Overview of the Recent Pharmaceutical Innovations. *Pharmaceutics*, 12(2), 142. http://dx.doi.org/10.3390/pharmaceutics12020142

Khan, I., Saeed, K., Khan, I. (2019). Nanoparticles: Properties, applications and toxicities, *Arabian Journal of Chemistry*, 12(7), 908-931, https://doi.org/10.1016/j.arabjc.2017.05.011.

Munir, M. U., Ahmed, A., Usman, M., & Salman, S. (2020). Recent Advances in Nanotechnology-Aided Materials in Combating Microbial Resistance and Functioning as Antibiotics Substitutes. *International journal of nanomedicine*, *15*, 7329–7358.

Natan, M., & Banin, E. (2017). From Nano to Micro: using nanotechnology to combat microorganisms and their multidrug resistance. *FEMS microbiology reviews*, *41*(3), 302–322. https://doi.org/10.1093/femsre/fux00

National Nanotechnology of Initiative (2021). Nano101, what it is and how it works. https://www.nano.gov/nanotech-101/what

Pelgrift, R. Y., & Friedman, A. J. (2013). Nanotechnology as a therapeutic tool to combat microbial resistance. *Advanced drug delivery reviews*, *65*(13-14), 1803–1815. https://doi.org/10.1016/j.addr.2013.07.011

Resistance mechanisms – Antibiotic resistance – ReAct. (2021). Retrieved 5 May 2021, from https://www.reactgroup.org/toolbox/understand/antibiotic-resistance/resistance-mechanisms-in-bacteria/

WHO (2020) Antibiotic resistance https://www.who.int/news-room/fact-sheets/detail/antibiotic-resistance

## *Chapter 7:*

Azam, H. A., & Tanji, Y. (2019). Bacteriophage-host arm race: an update on the mechanism of phage resistance in bacteria and revenge of the phage with the perspective for phage therapy. *Applied Microbiology and Biotechnology.*, *103*(5), 2121–2131. https://doi.org/10.1007/s00253-019-09629-x

Chan, K. B., Abedon, T. S., & Loc-Carrillo, C. (2013). Phage cocktails and the future of phage therapy. *Future Microbiology.*, *8*(6), 769–783. https://doi.org/10.2217/FMB.13.47

Ganeshan, S & Hosseinidoust, Z. (2019). Phage Therapy with a Focus on the Human Microbiota. *Antibiotics.*, *8*(3). https://doi.org/10.3390/antibiotics8030131

Hatfull, G. (2008). Bacteriophage genomics. *Current Opinion in Microbiology.*, *11*(5), 447–453. https://doi.org/10.1016/j.mib.2008.09.004

Hobbs, Z., & Abedon, T. S. (2016). Diversity of phage infection types and associated terminology: the problem with "Lytic or lysogenic". *FEMS Microbiology Letters.*, *363*(7). https://doi.org/10.1093/femsle/fnw047

Jariah, R., & Hakim, S. M. (2019). Interaction of phages, bacteria, and the human immune system: Evolutionary changes in phage therapy. *Reviews in Medical Virology.*, *29*(5). https://doi.org/10.1002/rmv.2055

Loc-Carrillo, C., & Abedon, T. S. (2011). Pros and cons of phage therapy. *Bacteriophage*, *1*(2), 111–114. https://doi.org/10.4161/bact.1.2.14590

Summers W. C. (2012). The strange history of phage therapy. *Bacteriophage*, *2*(2), 130–133. https://doi.org/10.4161/bact.20757

## *Chapter 8:*

Bartlett, J. G., Gilbert, D. N., & Spellberg, B. (2013). Seven ways to preserve the miracle of antibiotics. *Clinical Infectious Diseases: An Official Publication of the Infectious Diseases Society of America*, *56*(10), 1445–1450. https://doi.org/10.1093/cid/cit070

CDC. (2020, March 13). *What Exactly is Antibiotic Resistance?* Centers for Disease Control and Prevention. https://www.cdc.gov/drugresistance/about.html

Oliveira, J., & Reygaert, W. C. (2021). Gram Negative Bacteria. In *StatPearls*. StatPearls Publishing. http://

www.ncbi.nlm.nih.gov/books/NBK538213/

Simons, A., Alhanout, K., & Duval, R. E. (2020). Bacteriocins, Antimicrobial Peptides from Bacterial Origin: Overview of Their Biology and Their Impact against Multidrug-Resistant Bacteria. *Microorganisms*, *8*(5). https://doi.org/10.3390/microorganisms8050639

Sizar, O., & Unakal, C. G. (2021). Gram Positive Bacteria. In *StatPearls*. StatPearls Publishing. http://www.ncbi.nlm.nih.gov/books/NBK470553/

Soltani, S., Hammami, R., Cotter, P. D., Rebuffat, S., Said, L. B., Gaudreau, H., Bédard, F., Biron, E., Drider, D., & Fliss, I. (2021). Bacteriocins as a new generation of antimicrobials: Toxicity aspects and regulations. *FEMS Microbiology Reviews*, *45*(fuaa039). https://doi.org/10.1093/femsre/fuaa039

Ventola, C. L. (2015). The Antibiotic Resistance Crisis. *Pharmacy and Therapeutics*, *40*(4), 277–283.

Yang, S.-C., Lin, C.-H., Sung, C. T., & Fang, J.-Y. (2014). Antibacterial activities of bacteriocins: Application in foods and pharmaceuticals. *Frontiers in Microbiology*, *5*. https://doi.org/10.3389/fmicb.2014.00241

*Chapter 9:*

Afify, A. E., Baroty, G. S., Baz, F. K., Baky, H. H., & Murad, S. A. (2018). Scenedesmus obliquus: Antioxidant and antiviral activity of proteins hydrolyzed by three enzymes. *Journal of Genetic Engineering and Biotechnology, 16*(2), 399-408. doi:10.1016/j.jgeb.2018.01.002

Al-Judaibi, A. (2014). Antibacterial Effects of Extracts of Two Types of Red Sea Algae. *Journal of Biosciences and Medicines, 02*(02), 74-82. doi:10.4236/jbm.2014.22012

Alboofetileh, M., Rezaei, M., Tabarsa, M., Rittà, M., Donalisio, M., Mariatti, F., . . . Cravotto, G. (2019). Effect of different non-conventional extraction methods on the antibacterial and antiviral activity of fucoidans extracted from Nizamuddinia zanardinii. *International Journal of Biological Macromolecules, 124*, 131-137. doi:10.1016/j.ijbiomac.2018.11.201

Beaulieu, L., Bondu, S., Doiron, K., Rioux, L., & Turgeon, S. L. (2015). Characterization of antibacterial activity from protein hydrolysates of the macroalga Saccharina longicruris and identification of peptides implied in bioactivity. *Journal of Functional Foods, 17*, 685-697. doi:10.1016/j.jff.2015.06.026

Besednova, N. N., Andryukov, B. G., Zaporozhets, T. S., Kryzhanovsky, S. P., Kuznetsova, T. A., Fedyanina, L. N., . . . Zvyagintseva, T. N. (2020). Algae Polyphenolic Compounds and Modern Antibacterial Strategies: Current Achievements and Immediate Prospects. *Biomedicines, 8*(9), 342. doi:10.3390/biomedicines8090342

Besednova, N. N., Andryukov, B. G., Zaporozhets, T. S., Kryzhanovsky, S. P., Fedyanina, L. N., Kuznetsova, T. A., . . . Shchelkanov, M. Y. (2021). Antiviral Effects of Polyphenols

from Marine Algae. *Biomedicines, 9*(2), 200. doi:10.3390/
biomedicines9020200

Bhowmick, S., Mazumdar, A., Moulick, A., & Adam, V. (2020).
Algal metabolites: An inevitable substitute for antibiotics.
*Biotechnology Advances, 43*, 107571. doi:10.1016/
j.biotechadv.2020.107571

Reygaert, W.C. (2018). An overview of the antimicrobial
resistance mechanisms of bacteria. *AIMS Microbiology, 4*(3),
482–501. https://doi.org/10.3934/microbiol.2018.3.482

Catarino, M., Silva, A., & Cardoso, S. (2018). Phycochemical
Constituents and Biological Activities of Fucus spp. *Marine
Drugs, 16*(8), 249. doi:10.3390/md16080249

Cherian, C., Vennila, J. J., & Sharan, L. (2019). Marine
bromophenols as an effective inhibitor of virulent proteins
(peptidyl arginine deiminase, gingipain R and hemagglutinin A)
in Porphyromas gingivalis. *Archives of Oral Biology, 100*,
119-128. doi:10.1016/j.archoralbio.2019.02.016

Desbois, A. P., & Smith, V. J. (2009). Antibacterial free fatty
acids: Activities, mechanisms of action and biotechnological
potential. *Applied Microbiology and Biotechnology, 85*(6),
1629-1642. doi:10.1007/s00253-009-2355-3

He, F., Yang, Y., Yang, G., & Yu, L. (2010). Studies on
antibacterial activity and antibacterial mechanism of a novel
polysaccharide from Streptomyces virginia H03. *Food Control,
21*(9), 1257-1262. doi:10.1016/j.foodcont.2010.02.013

Holesh, J. E., Aslam, S., & Martin, A. (2020). Physiology, Carbohydrates. In StatPearls. StatPearls Publishing.

Hughes, C. C., & Fenical, W. (2010). Antibacterials from the Sea. *Chemistry – A European Journal, 16*(42), 12512-12525. doi:10.1002/chem.201001279

Irshad, M., Reijden, W. A., Crielaard, W., & Laine, M. L. (2012). In Vitro Invasion and Survival of Porphyromonas gingivalis in Gingival Fibroblasts; Role of the Capsule. *Archivum Immunologiae Et Therapiae Experimentalis, 60*(6), 469-476. doi:10.1007/s00005-012-0196-8

Kabara, J. J., Swieczkowski, D. M., Conley, A. J., & Truant, J. P. (1972). Fatty Acids and Derivatives as Antimicrobial Agents. *Antimicrobial Agents and Chemotherapy, 2*(1), 23-28. doi:10.1128/aac.2.1.23

Lefranc, F., Koutsaviti, A., Ioannou, E., Kornienko, A., Roussis, V., Kiss, R., & Newman, D. (2019). Algae metabolites: Fromin vitro growth inhibitory effects to promising anticancer activity. *Natural Product Reports, 36*(5), 810-841. doi:10.1039/c8np00057c

Lijun, H., Nianjun, X., Jiangong, S., Xiaojun, Y., & Chengkui, Z. (2005). Isolation and pharmacological activities of bromophenols fromRhodomela confervoides. *Chinese Journal of Oceanology and Limnology, 23*(2), 226-229. doi:10.1007/bf02894243

McKee, T., & McKee, J. R. (2021). *Biochemistry the molecular basis of life*. Oxford University Press.

Mittal, N., Tesfu, H. H., Hogan, A. M., Cardona, S. T., & Sorensen, J. L. (2019). Synthesis and antibiotic activity of novel acylated phloroglucinol compounds against methicillin-resistant Staphylococcus aureus. *The Journal of Antibiotics, 72*(5), 253-259. doi:10.1038/s41429-019-0153-4

Munita, J. M., & Arias, C. A. (2016). Mechanisms of Antibiotic Resistance. *Microbiology Spectrum, 4*(2), 3–37. https://doi.org/10.1128/microbiolspec.vmbf-0016-2015

National Center for Biotechnology Information (2021). PubChem Compound Summary for CID 359, Phloroglucinol. Retrieved May 6, 2021 from https://pubchem.ncbi.nlm.nih.gov/compound/Phloroglucinol.

National Geographic Society. (2012, October 09). Autotroph. Retrieved from https://www.nationalgeographic.org/encyclopedia/autotroph/#:~:text=Algae, which live in water,photosynthesis to make their food

Pandey, K. B., & Rizvi, S. I. (2009). Plant Polyphenols as Dietary Antioxidants in Human Health and Disease. *Oxidative Medicine and Cellular Longevity, 2*(5), 270-278. doi:10.4161/oxim.2.5.9498

Pantosti, A., & Venditti, M. (2009). What is MRSA? *European Respiratory Journal, 34*(5), 1190-1196. doi:10.1183/09031936.00007709

Parsaeimehr, A., & Lutzu, G. (2016). Algae as a Novel Source of Antimicrobial Compounds. *Antibiotic Resistance,* 377-396.

doi:10.1016/b978-0-12-803642-6.00018-6

Pratt, R., Daniels, T. C., Eiler, J. J., Gunnison, J. B., Kumler, W. D., Oneto, J. F., . . . Strain, H. H. (1944). Chlorellin, An Antibacterial Substance From Chlorella. *Science, 99*(2574), 351-352. doi:10.1126/science.99.2574.351

Pérez, M., Falqué, E., & Domínguez, H. (2016). Antimicrobial Action of Compounds from Marine Seaweed. *Marine Drugs, 14*(3), 52. doi:10.3390/md14030052

Rajauria, G., & Abu-Ghannam, N. (2013). Isolation and Partial Characterization of Bioactive Fucoxanthin fromHimanthalia elongataBrown Seaweed: A TLC-Based Approach. *International Journal of Analytical Chemistry, 2013*, 1-6. doi:10.1155/2013/802573

Reygaert, W. C. (2013, December 1). *Antimicrobial resistance mechanisms of Staphylococcus aureus*. ResearchGate. https://www.researchgate.net/publication/267695121_Antimicrobial_resistance_mechanisms_of_Staphylococcus_aureus

Shannon, E., & Abu-Ghannam, N. (2016). Antibacterial Derivatives of Marine Algae: An Overview of Pharmacological Mechanisms and Applications. *Marine Drugs, 14*(4), 81. doi:10.3390/md14040081

Silva, A., Silva, S. A., Carpena, M., Garcia-Oliveira, P., Gullón, P., Barroso, M. F., . . . Simal-Gandara, J. (2020). Macroalgae as a Source of Valuable Antimicrobial Compounds: Extraction and

Applications. *Antibiotics, 9*(10), 642. doi:10.3390/
antibiotics9100642

Taylor, T. A. (2020, August 23). Staphylococcus Aureus.
Retrieved from https://www.ncbi.nlm.nih.gov/books/
NBK441868/

Tsao, R. (2010). Chemistry and Biochemistry of Dietary
Polyphenols. *Nutrients, 2*(12), 1231-1246. doi:10.3390/
nu2121231

Wang, Y., et al. "Sensitivity of Escherichia coli to seaweed
(Ascophyllum nodosum) phlorotannins and terrestrial tannins."
Asian - Australasian Journal of Animal Sciences, 22(2), 238.
Gale Academic OneFile, link.gale.com/apps/doc/A195919162/
AONE?u=ocul_mcmaster&sid=AONE&xid=59c82b21.
Accessed 6 May 2021

Xu, S., Huang, X., & Cheong, K. (2017). Recent Advances in
Marine Algae Polysaccharides: Isolation, Structure, and
Activities. *Marine Drugs, 15*(12), 388. doi:10.3390/md15120388

## Chapter 10:

*Antimicrobial Stewardship*. Public Health Ontario. (2019,
October 22). https://www.publichealthontario.ca/en/health-
topics/antimicrobial-stewardship.

Bui, V. (2020, March). *Fighting COVID-19 starts with universal
access to water and sanitation.* The Council of Canadians.

https://canadians.org/analysis/fighting-covid-19-starts-universal-access-water-and-sanitation.

CDC. (2018, November 5). *One Health Basics*. Centers for Disease Control and Prevention. https://www.cdc.gov/onehealth/basics/index.html#:~:text=One%20Health%20is%20a%20collaborative,plants%2C%20and%20their%20shared%20environment

Davis, C. P. (2020, October 6). *What's a Virus? Viral Infection Types, Symptoms, Treatment*. OnHealth. https://www.onhealth.com/content/1/viral_infections#:~:text=What%20Is%20a%20Viral%20Infection,to%20make%20more%20virus%20particles

Government of Canada, S. C. (2019, June 17). *Visible Minority (15), Individual Low-income Status (6), Low-income Indicators (4), Generation Status (4), Age (6) and Sex (3) for the Population in Private Households of Canada, Provinces and Territories, Census Metropolitan Areas and Census Agglomerations, 2016 Census - 25% Sample Data*. Statistics Canada. https://www12.statcan.gc.ca/census-recensement/2016/dp-pd/dt-td/Rp-eng.cfm?TABID=2&Lang=E&APATH=3&DETAIL=0&DIM=0&FL=A&FREE=0&GC=0&GID=1341679&GK=0&GRP=1&PID=110563&PRID=10&PTYPE=109445&S=0&SHOWALL=0&SUB=0&Temporal=2017&THEME=120&VID=0&VNAMEE=&VNAMEF=&D1=0&D2=0&D3=0&D4=0&D5=0&D6=0

*Hand Hygiene and Antibiotic Resistance*. Minnesota Dept. of Health. (2019, November 25). https://www.health.state.mn.us/

people/handhygiene/why/resistance.html

Henkel Canada. (2020, July 22). *Canadian Survey Shows Handwashing Habits Have Significantly Changed Since COVID-19*. Cision Canada. https://www.newswire.ca/news-releases/canadian-survey-shows-handwashing-habits-have-significantly-changed-since-covid-19-813135590.html

McKenna, M. (n.d.). *Covid-19 May Worsen the Antibiotic Resistance Crisis*. Wired. https://www.wired.com/story/covid-19-may-worsen-the-antibiotic-resistance-crisis/

Mills, O. (2020, September 20). *Connecting Water and Hygiene Expertise With Need In a Smaller World*. Centre for Affordable Water and Sanitation Technology (CAWST). https://www.cawst.org/about/news/cawstinthenews/2020/09/connecting-water-and-hygiene-expertise-with-need-in-a-smaller-world/

Sagren, M. (2021, February 15). *How COVID-19 is Shaping Antibiotic Resistance*. Science in the News. https://sitn.hms.harvard.edu/flash/2021/how-covid-19-is-shaping-antibiotic-resistance/#:~:text=Containment%20of%20COVID%2D19%20within,resistant%20infections%20especially%20within%20hospitals

Strathdee, S. A., Davies, S. C., & Marcelin, J. R. (2020). Confronting Antimicrobial Resistance Beyond the COVID-19 Pandemic and the 2020 US Election. *The Lancet, 396*(10257), 1050–1053. https://doi.org/10.1016/s0140-6736(20)32063-8

Subedi, R., Greenberg, T. L., & Turcotte, M. (2020, October 28). *COVID-19 Mortality Rates in Canada's Ethno-cultural Neighbourhoods*. Statistics Canada. https://www150.statcan.gc.ca/n1/pub/45-28-0001/2020001/article/00079-eng.htm

Zhou, F., Yu, T., Du, R., Fan, G., Liu, Y., Liu, Z., … Cao, B. (2020). Clinical Course and Risk Factors for Mortality of Adult Inpatients with COVID-19 in Wuhan, China: A Retrospective Cohort Study. *The Lancet*, *395*(10229), 1054–1062. https://doi.org/10.1016/s0140-6736(20)30566-3

www.ingramcontent.com/pod-product-compliance
Lightning Source LLC
Chambersburg PA
CBHW061742270326
41928CB00011B/2337